THE
HEALING
INTELLIGENCE
OF
ESSENTIAL OILS

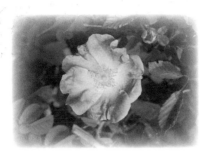

"Dr. Schnaubelt shows a cutting-edge aromatherapy perspective in this book and gives us many answers to deeply understand the co-evolution of plants and human beings."

AYAKO BERG, LONDON SCHOOL OF AROMATHERAPY, JAPAN

"Kurt Schnaubelt continues his professional validation of essential oils as serious health care products. Using in-depth but approachable science, Schnaubelt shows how humans and plants have evolved together, supporting and influencing each other's development and well-being over millennia. Each section of this beautifully illustrated book covers a different area of aromatherapy study, from how to recognize authentic oils to recipes for basic health issues and all interspersed with delightful "Essential Oil Journeys" that trace the use of plant essences around the world. Suitable for professional therapists of all kinds while still accessible to the home practitioner, *The Healing Intelligence of Essential Oils* is destined to become a well-thumbed classic in every health library."

SUZANNE CATTY, AUTHOR OF *HYDROSOLS:*
THE NEXT AROMATHERAPY

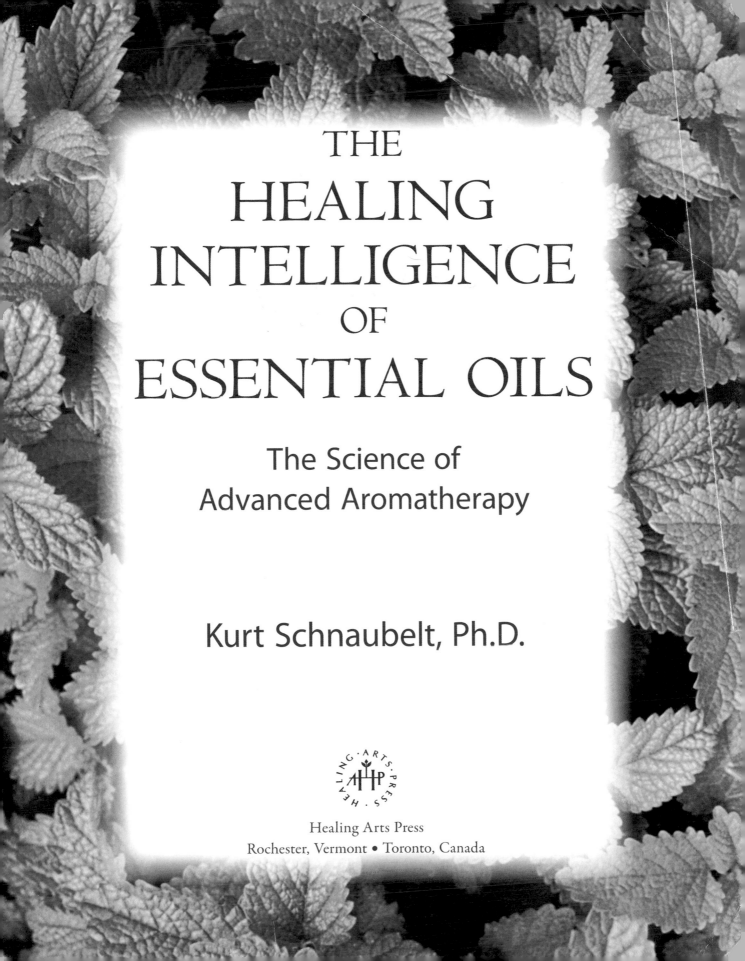

THE
HEALING
INTELLIGENCE
OF
ESSENTIAL OILS

The Science of
Advanced Aromatherapy

Kurt Schnaubelt, Ph.D.

Healing Arts Press
Rochester, Vermont • Toronto, Canada

Healing Arts Press
One Park Street
Rochester, Vermont 05767
www.HealingArtsPress.com

Healing Arts Press is a division of Inner Traditions International

*Note to the reader: This book is intended as an informational guide. The remedies,
approaches, and techniques described herein are meant to supplement, and not to be a
substitute for, professional medical care or treatment. They should not be used to treat
a serious ailment without prior consultation with a qualified health care professional.*

Library of Congress Cataloging-in-Publication Data
Schnaubelt, Kurt.
  The healing intelligence of essential oils : the science of advanced aromatherapy /
Kurt Schnaubelt.
      p. cm.
  Includes bibliographical references and index.
  Summary: "Explores science's new biological understanding of essential oils
for improved immunity and treatment of degenerative diseases"— Provided by
publisher.
  ISBN 978-1-59477-425-6 (pbk.) — ISBN 978-1-59477-815-5 (e-book)
  1. Aromatherapy. I. Title.
  RM666.A68S364 2011
  615.3'219—dc23

                                                                    2011023569

Printed and bound in India by Replika Press Pvt. Ltd.

10 9 8 7 6 5 4 3 2 1

Text design and layout by Priscilla Baker
This book was typeset in Garamond Premier Pro with Centaur and Myriad Pro
used as display typefaces

Unless otherwise noted, all photography and graphics by Monika Haas and Kurt
Schnaubelt

To send correspondence to the author of this book, mail a first-class letter to the
author c/o Inner Traditions • Bear & Company, One Park Street, Rochester, VT
05767, and we will forward the communication, or contact the author directly at
www.pacificinstituteofaromatherapy.com.

CONTENTS

INTRODUCTION

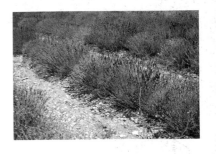

Spices provided the major incentive for voyaging into the unknown.

JOHN KEAY

The initial impulse to learn about aromatherapy is almost always instinctual. Courses, instructors, and books satisfy this impulse, yet learning about aromatherapy and using essential oils almost always turns into a dynamic process. It generally begins with a little experimentation, such as using oils for relaxation or a herpes treatment. With a little luck there is some success and we feel encouraged to continue. If we are open-minded and not too dependent (physically, mentally, or psychologically) on conventional drugs, we notice that taking care of common ailments with essential oils and other natural means leads to a state of better health.

In the best case, the process of using essential oils leads to a state in which we have enough self-confidence to maintain our own health without continuously consulting the conventional medical machine. Conventional medicine, with its technology and drugs, is something we generally use when we think we must, when we think that more natural ways are not sufficiently effective. Indeed, it has crucial benefits under certain circumstances. But at the same time, we know it is as overdone and self-defeating as a Ferrari without gasoline. It disempowers us if we attach too much of our well-being to it.

So it is a real advantage when we eventually reach sufficient equanimity and inner peace to know when to consult the conventional system and when to rely on ourselves and on natural healing instead. There is no substitute for cultivating an understanding of the natural way our soul and body works and how that precious natural balance can be maintained.

One of the barriers to our gaining that understanding arises from our cultural norms, which have made us worried about essential oils.

UNDERSTANDING AROMATHERAPY

Aromatherapy is not a luxury. It is an inexpensive way to maintain health and to treat many diseases naturally.

They are seen as potentially too strong, but nevertheless we are concerned they will fail us when challenged by serious conditions. Somehow we think "medicine" when we think of essential oils. We think of doctors who disapprove.

But we can be guided by remembering that there are other plant products to which we have developed a more relaxed relation, such as tea, made by steeping the leaves of *Camellia sinensis* in hot water. And what diversity there is in tea: Ceylon, Assam, Darjeeling, Japanese, Oolong, Ti Kuan Yin, Keemun, and so on. The list is long and tea enthusiasts know that all these teas taste different and have wildly different physiological effects. The dramatic health benefits of green tea are acknowledged without controversy, probably because nobody ever wrote a book called "teatherapy."

But just like we will not discover the wonderful varieties of tea if we stay with English Breakfast tea bags forever, we will not discover the true benefits of essential oils unless we explore the real beauty that lies in their authenticity. As we are inspired to explore essential oils more deeply, it is natural that we do so in ways that correspond to our use of conventional medicines. Connecting the old with the new, we begin to use antibacterial oils instead of antibiotics, because research shows that some essential oils are indeed effective against pathogenic bacteria. By using them we begin to avoid the negative side effects of antibiotics—a crucial step to better health, as it leads to a significantly improved immune response. As we move along, more questions arise. A crucial question in aromatherapy is what those essential oils really are.

Here we are constricted by another of the ways in which our culture stifles the experience of refined and complex natural products: the conceptual reduction of everything to one—generally bad—substance or culprit. Some will say they cannot drink tea because they cannot drink caffeine. Similarly wine is dismissed as "alcohol." As a consequence we often remain stuck with grossly simplified concepts of tea or wine—or, for that matter, essential oils. This is also reflected in the way these products are homogenized by industrial production. Instead of allowing the enormous variety in flavor and effect that nature presents, white wine in California is made to taste uniformly "fruity," no matter what the label claims. Instead of presenting an opportunity to enjoy the breadth of essential oil diversity, the bulk of Rosemary essential oil on offer is a standardized liquid engineered to cost no more than $45 a pound.

This book offers a unique approach by providing the vital context for the use of essential oils revealed by the new insights about aromatherapy arising today, mainly from the different branches of biology. In particular, discoveries about the origin of the physiological activity of plant substances have been very illuminating. Essential oils provide the most benefits for those who like to live in harmony with nature and find moderation and humility vis-à-vis creation desirable. Like exploring the world of tea, we can experience the refinement and finesse of essential oils instead of constantly talking about their potential hazards.

One of the ways to explore is to read books that tell us what to do with oils and what not to do. In the past, aromatherapy texts mainly instructed an aromatherapist on how she or he should practice. The aim of this book is to make it easier for the lay individual to self-medicate with essential oils. This individualized form of aromatherapy focuses more on exploring essential oil efficacy and less on formulating claims. This book aims to present this—almost underground—form of personal aromatherapy with its stunning benefits.

It will also highlight the continuously evolving scientific proof for new therapeutic possibilities.

How to Use this Book

Part 1, "Understanding the Language of Plants: The Science of Aromatherapy," presents an entirely new take on the theory of aromatherapy, exploring recent findings at the interface of evolutionary biology, cellular biology, and pharmacology, shedding light on the enormous importance the particular plant substances known as secondary metabolites* have for human health. These findings also highlight so far unrecognized qualities of multicomponent mixtures, such as essential oils, which hold distinct advantages over single component substances, such as drugs.

Part 2, "Exploring Authentic Essential Oils: Recognizing Authenticity, Safety, Diversity, Fragrance," offers guidelines for determining the authenticity of an essential oil and establishes the importance of using authentic oils. It also addresses the mostly false warnings about risks associated with the use of essential oils, while at the same time clearly noting the few areas of real concern and providing techniques for safe

---

*Please refer to the BioPrimer for a definition of this and other specialized biological terms.

use. Presentations of the diverse influences that have shaped aromatherapy offer insights into its efficacy. You will also find hints for actualizing an aromatherapy lifestyle. Finally, part 2 explores the role played by fragrance.

If you are in need of a remedy, you can turn directly to part 3, "Healing with Essential Oils: Treatment Strategies and Protocols," to discover which essential oils have been found helpful for specific conditions, and ways to apply them. The recipes range from topical and internal applications, to the use of essential oils in easing side effects of conventional cancer treatment and hepatitis, to suggestions derived from Chinese medicine for treatment of autoimmune diseases.

Accompanying the text throughout you will also find "Essential Oil Journeys" to guide your personal exploration of essential oils; each journey will connect you to one or more essential oils and the cultural diversity of the plant-human interface in which they have flourished.

In addition to the primary text in the center columns of this book, you will also find related short topics in the side panels. The side panels and boxes are divided into six categories, which are color-coded:

- **PLANTS IN ARTS AND CULTURE:** Humans have always connected with plants on many different planes. The purely medicinal approach to plants, essential oils, and aromatherapy is rather self-limiting. To free the study of aromatherapy from the exclusive rule of dry data we shall visit examples of the many different ways in which plants have been, and still are, part of culture, ritual, and religion.

- **SCIENTIFIC CONTEXT:** The main text moves forward quite quickly. These scientific side panels and boxes develop topics and offer helpful illustrations. They also refer to some of the books that deepen the subject matter in a fashion easily accessible to the lay reader or present abstracts from actual scientific papers to illustrate the form in which such results are originally communicated. Some of the common terms referring to the molecular makeup and physical properties of essential oils are also introduced in these panels.

- **CONTRIBUTORS TO AROMATHERAPY:** These side panels will introduce you to some of the individuals who have contributed to the foundations and the development of aromatherapy in ways that are at times not immediately obvious from the existing literature.

- **BACKGROUND INFORMATION:** The background panels present arguments or facts providing an added layer of context to the topics in the main narrative.
- **UNDERSTANDING AROMATHERAPY:** These side panels elaborate aspects of the main text directly related to the practice of aromatherapy.
- **RECIPE:** Specific recipes for essential oil blends are provided in these boxes.

At the end of the book you will find a section on valuable aromatherapy resources. As there are many excellent suppliers of essential oils and also of aromatherapy education, it is beyond the scope of this book to provide a comprehensive list of all suppliers. The resources section does include vendors of essential oils and education providers who share some of the basic ideas put forward in this book about essential oil authenticity and an approach to aromatherapy that recognizes the biological qualities of essential oils in addition to their chemical composition.

Important Note

Everything that is said in this book about the potential physiological and therapeutic qualities of essential oils pertains *only* to authentic essential oils.

As a result, the reader may find that French and European essential oils are mentioned more frequently than those from other places. The reason for this is part historic and part economic. Of course authentic essential oils can be produced all over the planet. However, only in France and some regions around the Mediterranean can artisanal distillers make a (modest) living by producing essential oils exclusively for use in aromatherapy. This is the reason that specialties such as the chemotypes of Thyme, the *decumbens* variety of Hyssop, or simply *Helichrysum italicum* mostly originate in France.

In the case of essential oils from the global, industrial "drive the price down" economy, the likelihood of becoming subject to the everyday deception inherent in almost all industrial products increases exponentially.

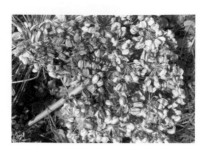

BIOPRIMER
Relevant Concepts and Terms

This book introduces a number of terms and concepts from the disciplines of biology and chemistry, which may not be very common in aromatherapy discourse. To facilitate reading of the book, the most essential terms are introduced together here. In addition, a more comprehensive glossary is provided at the end of the book for your reference.

Terms Relating to the Origin of Physiological Activity of Plant Substances

Two main categories of plant substances have been distinguished: primary and secondary metabolites.

> *Primary metabolites or primary plant substances* are all those components that comprise the bulk of the biomass and basically perform a plant's daily activities. They are proteins, carbohydrates, fats and oils, and genetic materials such as DNA.
>
> *Secondary metabolites* are substances that are spun off the biosynthetic pathways that manufacture primary metabolites, and then, coincidentally, help the survival of the plant (for instance, by repelling herbivores). Over time these substances became not only the defense mechanism but also the communication system of the plant. Essential oils are one large group of secondary plant metabolites (others are, for instance, alkaloids or even the dyes in the petals of flowers). For medicinal purposes, secondary metabolites attract the most interest.

Constituents of Essential Oils

Essential oils have two main categories of constituents: one category is that of the terpenes; the other category is that of the phenylpropanes.

Terpenes are the largest group of components found in the essential oils of plants. These organic compounds are major biosynthetic building blocks within nearly every living creature. Terpenes have historically been classified by the number of terpene units in the molecule, indicated by a prefix in the name, giving rise to mono-terpenes, sesquiterpenes, diterpenes, and so on. The term is used sometimes more narrowly and sometimes more broadly in the lay as well as the scientific literature. Strictly speaking, terpenes are hydrocarbon molecules with ten carbon atoms and a varying number of hydrogen atoms. However *terpenes* is generally used as an umbrella term, which includes terpene molecules that have been modified by the introduction of oxygen. The unifying concept of the broader use of the term *terpenes* is biological in origin, as the above components all arise from a common biosynthetic pathway that builds terpenes, sesquiterpenes, and ultimately steroids and cholesterol.

Phenylpropanoids, the other major group of components in essential oils, are found throughout the plant kingdom, where they serve as essential components of a number of structural polymers. Among other things, phenylpropanoid derivatives, such as floral pigments and fragrant compounds, provide protection from ultraviolet light, defend against herbivores and pathogens, and mediate plant-pollinator interactions. Phenylpropanes are distinguished by their biosynthetic origin, ultimately arising from amino acid synthesis in the chloroplast.

Solubility and Polarity

The distinguishing physical characteristic of essential oils is their *lipophilic* nature.

Lipophilic means "oily or oil soluble, water insoluble."
Hydrophilic means "water soluble."

Polarity is the property in chemistry and physics that makes molecules either lipophilic or hydrophilic.

If electrons are equally shared in the chemical bonds of a molecule, the molecule is *nonpolar,* causing it to assume an oily character and making it less or not at all soluble in water. *Polarity* arises when the electrons in a chemical bond are not shared equally. This results in increased solubility in water. The terms *polar* and *water soluble* are therefore often used interchangeably, as are *nonpolar* and *lipophilic.*

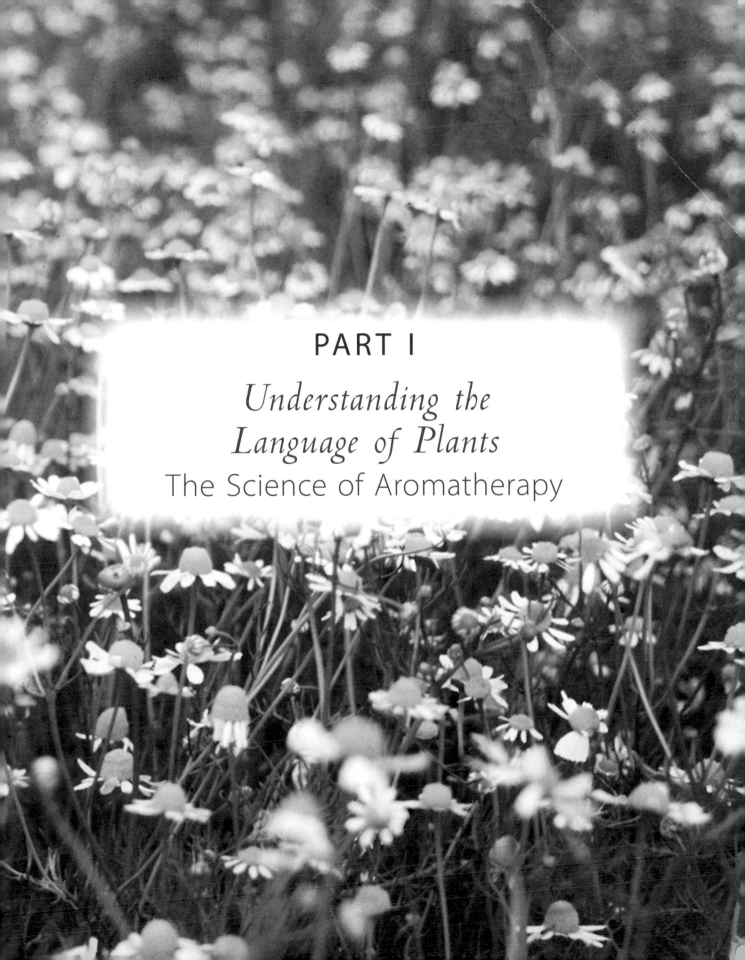

PART I

Understanding the Language of Plants
The Science of Aromatherapy

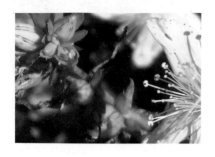

ONE

THE FOUNDATIONS OF AROMATHERAPY

Oil of Lavender, when made by passing flowers through a glass alembic, surpasses all other perfumes.

DIOSCORIDES, *DE MATERIA MEDICA*

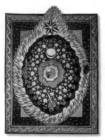

What Is an Essential Oil?

Looking to the origin of the word *essence* is instructive. It can be traced to the ancient and medieval *quintessence*. For Plato *quintessence* represented that of which the cosmos itself is made. In the Middle Ages *quintessence* meant the fifth element beyond earth, water, fire, and air. Throughout the Middle Ages the words *essence, quintessence,* or *essential oil* also represented the various degrees of refinement associated with distillation. The process of evaporating an often hazy and less-than-pure liquid into an essentially invisible gaseous form and the subsequent condensation of the steam into a clear and fragrant, obviously pure, distillate must have evoked these notions. Hence the essence, the distillate, was always invested with qualities beyond the material, ranging from the esoteric to the spiritual.

With the ascent of chemistry in the late nineteenth and early twentieth century came the demystification and much broader availability of the distillation process. Essential oils began to be seen as the result of a clever technological process. The all-encompassing avalanche of reductionism (in which complex phenomena are explained by parsing them down to ever smaller components and then analyzing the simplest, most basic physical mechanisms present) mercilessly devoured the hitherto magical essences and turned them into oily or oil soluble (lipophilic) mobile liquids, derived from plants by steam distillation. The advances in chemical analysis made it possible to understand essential oils as, often complex, mixtures of substances.

Not surprisingly, the first book on aromatherapy was published in 1937 by a chemist in the employ of a perfume company: René-Maurice Gattefossé's *Aromathérapie*.[1] The tenor of the book was to espouse the healing properties of essential oils and to explain those healing properties as a quality of the molecules that had thus far been detected in essential oils.

Exploring Essential Oil Activity the Conventional Way

Aromatherapy has been strongly influenced by two core issues that have been in plain sight since its modern resurgence, yet their defining character has barely been recognized. One issue shaping aromatherapy is the apparent diversity of philosophical and scientific approaches that contribute to the healing strategies of aromatherapy, which will be discussed in detail in chapter 6. Another is the desire to convince the medical mainstream of the benefits of essential oil treatment. To satisfy this desire, scientific explanations for physiological and pharmacological efficacy of essential oils have remained in high demand.

However, in contemporary culture, only a very narrow form of conventional pharmacological proof qualifies as valid science. This leads to unexpected questions. For example, the attempt to explain the benefits of Lavender essential oil quickly turns into an exercise in epistemology. As we experience Lavender's outstanding capacity to heal burns, we wonder why we cannot claim this as a valid property. Then we notice that there is no research on this topic. And then we notice that the absence of research gives rise to the contention that Lavender is ineffective.

This unsatisfactory status quo is propagated as the mainstream dialogue equates reductionist chemistry and physics with science per se, ignoring other scientific approaches better suited to describing the physiological efficacy of natural extracts. As a consequence, real phenomena that evade description with the language of reductionism are ignored.

It is a defining problem of conventional medicine that realities that defy reductionist interpretation are treated as nonexistent. In silent

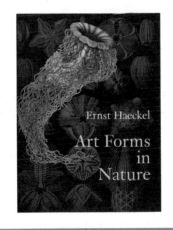

conspiracy, the industry acts as if such phenomena simply do not exist: "It is impossible that Lavender heals burns, because there is no research."

Why Pharmacology Cannot Demonstrate Essential Oil Efficacy

To demonstrate the effect of a synthetic drug or a natural substance within the framework of pharmacology, two conditions need to be fulfilled. First, there needs to be an experiment connecting a specific substance to a specific effect. For example, to ascertain whether or not the molecule citral is a sedative, the duration of induced sleep in test animals is measured. In an ideal experiment, a specific amount of citral puts the test animal to sleep for a specific duration of time. If the dosage of citral is increased, the sleep duration would then be correspondingly longer.

Second, pharmacology expects to see the results of its experiments fit into a larger narrative, which describes a mechanism for the observed action. For instance, citral acts as a sedative, because it decreases the irritability of the central nervous system. Ideally this contention is then demonstrated by another experiment, this time with a model on a lower level of organization, that is, not subjecting the whole animal to the test drug but showing the influence of citral on isolated nerve tissue.

The Reductionist Limitation

In a reductionist experiment only one of all possible variables is allowed to change. All others have to be kept at a constant value. This standard reductionist process works relatively well for single component drugs, such as aspirin. In the case of essential oils—where there is a potentially very large number of components contributing to the curative effect—this process is elusive, as the same experiment would then have to be repeated for each component of the essential oil. While this might then be a proper reductionist procedure, it is neither practically possible nor would it describe a meaningful reality.

In order to make statements about multicomponent mixtures, pharmacology is forced to pick a (presumed) active ingredient and to measure its effect, if for no other reason than to keep the number of experiments manageable. One has to conclude that the active ingredi-

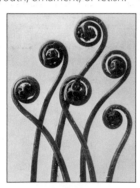

ent concept does not arise from observing specific activity but is instead maintained so the reductionist process makes sense.

Using Lavender as a remedy for burns is again the classic example. It is highly effective, but only within the aromatherapy community. Pharmacology does not recommend the use of Lavender, since it cannot find an active ingredient that mimics the effect of the whole oil.

Classic Research

To prepare for our foray into the biological explanations of essential oil efficacy we shall first review some important examples of the therapeutic or curative effects of essential oils that *have,* despite the limitations just outlined, been recognized through conventional reductionist experimentation. This section is purposely kept brief, as basically all of this has been extensively discussed in the literature. Still, it shows that—despite the lack of corporate interest—a sound body of knowledge about verifiable effects of essential oils was compiled even before cellular and evolutionary biology revealed the new dimensions of aromatherapy knowledge, which we will explore in detail in chapters 2 and 3.

Antibacterial Activity

The antibacterial activity of essential oils has continuously been researched since the 1880s. Their efficacy against many bacterial pathogens has been demonstrated in countless in vitro experiments. Gattefossé's book has a long list of references to such studies beginning as early as the late 1800s. These studies suggest that essential oils either inhibit bacterial growth or kill the bacteria outright. Possibly the most comprehensive studies were performed by Paul Belaiche in the 1970s.[2] The language barrier has provided an excuse for many anglophonic guardians of pharmacological orthodoxy to act as if these studies never happened.

While antibacterial efficacy of essential oils was demonstrated in petri dish experiments, its mechanism could not be explained with a square reductionist argument. Unlike antibiotics, which are active due to inhibiting an easily identifiable single target, the activity of essential oils, impairing a bacterium in multiple physiological systems as well as in membrane functionality, is only now understood (see chapter 2).

SCIENTIFIC CONTEXT
Hildebert Wagner

Hildebert Wagner was professor of pharmaceutical biology at Munich's Ludwig Maximilian University for more than thirty years. He published key studies on the spasmolytic and sedative qualities of essential oils. Together with Norman Farnsworth and Xiao Pei Gen, Hildebert Wagner represents the dramatic advances of pharmacognosy (the study of medicines derived from natural sources) in the 1970s.

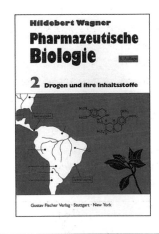

The Foundations of Aromatherapy

Absolutes vs. Essential Oils

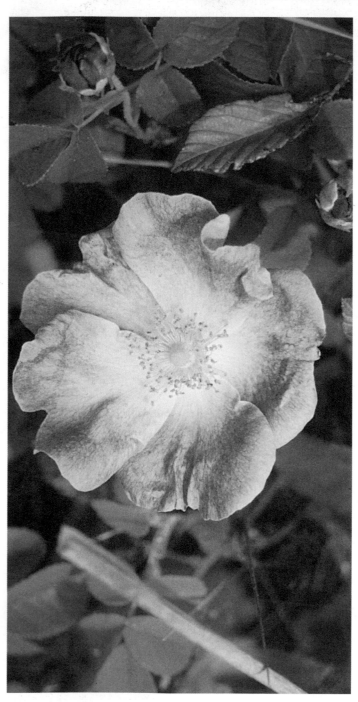

Rosa gallica, with its inimitable, most sublime fragrance

What better example to explore the difference between an essential oil and an absolute than Rose! Absolute production from *Rosa centifolia* is prevalent in Morocco, whereas *Rosa damascena* is primarily distilled in Turkey and Bulgaria, but also in Iran and parts of the former Soviet Union.

The differences in chemical composition between the essential oil and the absolute are well researched. A substantial concentration of phenyl ethyl alcohol is present in the absolute, yet only very little in the essential oil. The difference in fragrance is dramatic. Absolutes have a considerably more complex composition than essential oils, which is a consequence of their production by extraction. To end up in the extract, a plant molecule only needs to dissolve; there is no need to evaporate. Molecules that do not readily evaporate are not found in essential oils but may well end up in an absolute. Pragmatically, absolutes are mostly used—as indicated by their usually rather lofty prices—for luxurious perfumery.

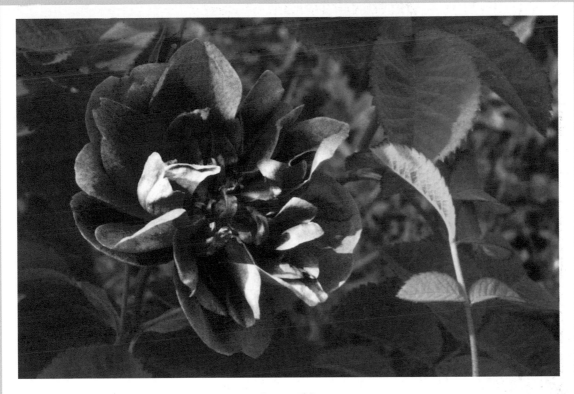

Rosa centifolia

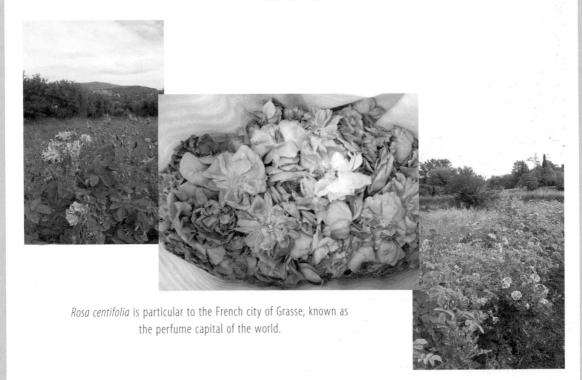

Rosa centifolia is particular to the French city of Grasse, known as the perfume capital of the world.

CONTRIBUTORS TO AROMATHERAPY

Paul Belaiche

Paul Belaiche determined the activity of over forty essential oils vis-à-vis pathogens encountered in common infections: *Proteus morgani, Proteus mirabilis, Proteus rettgeri* (intestinal), *Alcalescens dispar, Corynebacterium xerosa* (diphteria), *Neisseria flava* (sinus and ears), *Klebsiella pneumoniae* (pneumonia), *Staphylococcus alba* (food poisoning), *Staphylococcus aureus* (wounds), *Pneumococcus,* and *Candida albicans.*

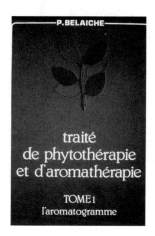

Antifungal Activity

Classical studies were conducted in the 1960s by J. C. Maruzella[3] and in the 1970s by J. Pellecuer.[4] Essential oil efficacy against fungi and yeasts has been demonstrated in vitro, but again, no mechanisms have been derived from these experiments. It was shown in the 1990s that the sterol insensitive key enzyme HMG CoA reductase in fungi can be inhibited by essential oils (see chapter 13).

Anti-inflammative Activity

Classic studies on the anti-inflammative effects of Chamomile (*Matricaria recutita*) were published in the 1980s.[5] Many sesquiterpene hydrocarbon components of essential oils have been demonstrated to have anti-inflammative effects on tissue. While the cellular and biochemical mechanisms are not clearly understood, sesquiterpene hydrocarbons have an obvious capacity to dissipate free radicals, the agents of inflammation.

Antiviral Activity

In the first sixty years of the twentieth century, viral diseases were not as well understood as they are today, and they were culturally overshadowed by bacterial infections. Human industriousness had created effective antibiotics for bacterial infections. For viral diseases there was . . . nothing.

The beginning of the AIDS crisis established the concept of a virus as something radically different from a bacterium in the public consciousness. This was also the time that the absence of industrial antiviral drugs was noticed. However, for those open to plant medicine, essential oils came to the rescue.

In 1987 Lembke and Deininger published their groundbreaking study about antiviral (and also antibacterial and antifungal) properties of essential oils and their components.[6] Many more studies followed worldwide, corroborating their findings. Today, this study seems prescient as it foreshadowed the recognition of nonselective effects. The efficacy of many oils and their components against a wide range of viruses has been demonstrated in vitro and occasionally in clinical trials. Different cellular mechanisms for the observations have been proposed.[7] The stunning efficacy of all or almost all essential oils against herpes lesions is probably the best example for a curious mind to experience the true meaning of nonselective effects first hand.

Anti-inflammative Chamomile

German Chamomile is distilled in many places, from South Africa and Nepal to Egypt and Chile. It is cultivated and distilled in Central Europe, for instance in Germany, Hungary, and Slovenia. Much research has gone into the selection and breeding of Chamomile plants with a particularly high content of alpha bisabolol, or more precisely (-)-alpha-bisabolol, the main anti-inflammative component of the essential oil.

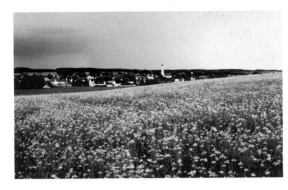

German Chamomile cultivation north of Munich

Alpha bisabolol is a delicate sesquiterpene alcohol component that is oxidized as the plant ages. The resulting bisabolol oxide or bisabolone-type essential oils are not as desirable for aromatherapy as the (-)-alpha-bisabolol type. An authentic essential oil of the (-)-alpha-bisabolol type will display a broad spectrum of effects that make it one of the most valuable essential oils.

The essential oil of German Chamomile is a powerful anti-inflammative when used topically; it soothes gastric pain when a drop is added to Chamomile tea. The French literature says it detoxifies bacterial waste products during and after infectious diseases and recent research credits it as a rare agent effective in the relief of COPD, chronic obstructive pulmonary disease.

Essential oil of German Chamomile is completely nontoxic and nonirritating and serves as a welcome universally applicable agent to reduce ever-present inflammative processes. Addition of German Chamomile essential oil to face and body oils always works.

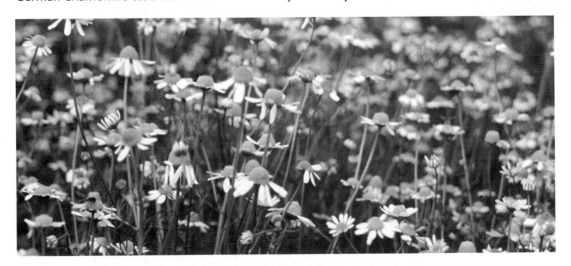

German Chamomile

North America: Tea Tree and Monarda

Tea Tree oil has received wide distribution as a nail fungus remedy and an addition to shampoo. It is a safe and commonly used antimicrobial agent even outside the aromatherapy community.

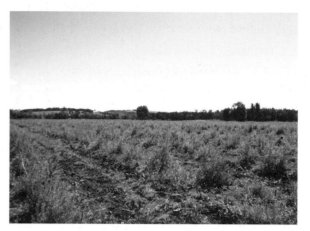

Tea Tree Plantation in Ballina, NSW. Tea Tree is every farmer's dream, as it grows without needing too much attention, and when the plants are at an appropriate height they are cut off with a combine, only to grow back without much ado.

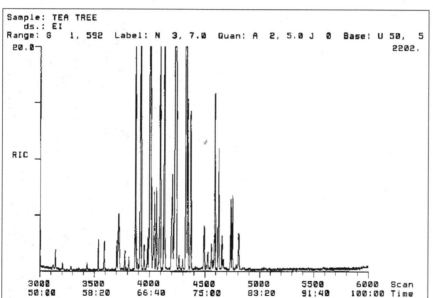

```
Sample: TEA TREE
    ds.: EI
Range: G  1, 592  Label: N  3, 7.0  Quan: A  2, 5.0 J  0  Base: U 50,  5
 20.0                                                            2202.



RIC




       3000      3500      4000      4500      5000      5500      6000  Scan
       50:00     58:20     66:40     75:00     83:20     91:40    100:00 Time
```

Once the essential oil is distilled, the value of the oil is documented with analysis, showing that the right components are present in the appropriate concentrations.

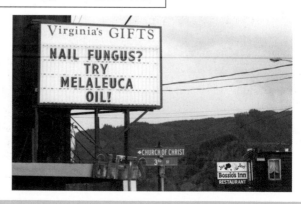

Scene from rural Oregon

On the other end of the spectrum is *Monarda fistulosa* from Quebec, an aromatherapy specialty. It has a brilliant fragrance and, for most individuals, leaves a slightly sharp but pleasant tingle on the skin when used in the shower. It is one of the most effective antiviral essential oils and is effective for upper respiratory and urogenital infections.

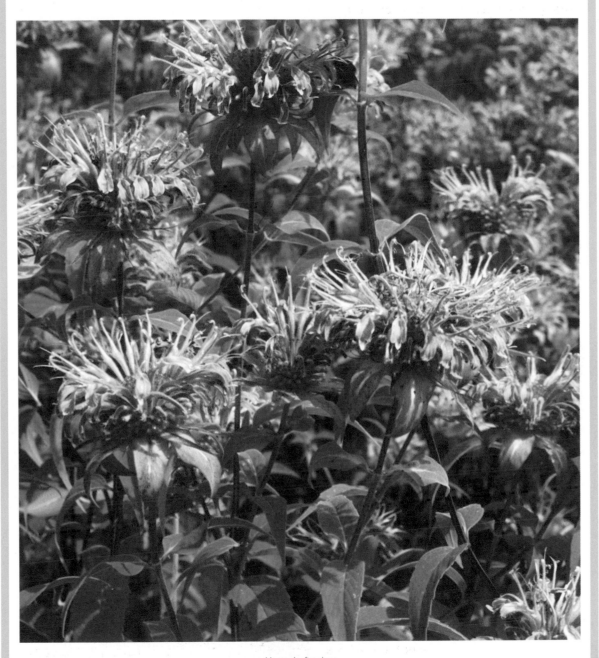

Monarda fistulosa

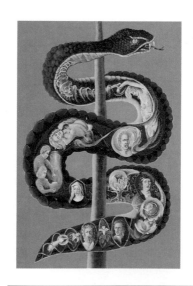
Effects Mediated via the Autonomic Nervous System

Classic studies were published by H. Wagner in 1973, in which spasmolytic (relieving cramps, spasms, and convulsions) and sedative effects were shown for essential oils in different pharmacological models.[8] The ability of essential oils to release or ameliorate anxiety, heart palpitations, nervousness, and heat flashes was demonstrated in double blind studies in the 1970s.

Recent Developments

In the middle of the twentieth century, an accumulation of data on essential oil pharmacology was afforded by the experimental methods of the time. There was a strong emphasis on antimicrobial activity and also on effects that can be characterized by measuring tone or tension in muscle or nerve tissue.

Then, as more refined methods became available in the 1980s and 1990s, the effects of essential oils on chronic, metabolic, and hormonal diseases were recognized. In the late 1990s there was a proliferation of research on the antitumor effects of terpenoid and also other essential oil components. Research had already progressed to successful clinical trials. Then, in 2001, all of a sudden the research stopped. Why this promising development was not pursued more vigorously, and was apparently even abandoned, is anybody's guess. It does not appear too outlandish to suspect reservations on the part of corporate pharmacology about remedies that might be too cheap and too accessible.

As physiological activity was discovered for a growing number of essential oil components, the active ingredient concept was expanded to allow for multiple active components and for resulting synergistic effects. But whenever a new type of activity was reported, the most common terpene molecules were implicated again and again as the responsible substances. From antiviral and antitumor to influencing the calcium uptake, ubiquitous compounds like linalool and limonene were credited with a growing portfolio of pharmacological properties. Assuming that an active ingredient produces only one or two specific effects was simply no longer describing the reality that could be observed.

Nonetheless, scientific understanding of essential oil activity remained based on variations of the active ingredient concept. And in

SCIENTIFIC CONTEXT

Abstract of the Original Study on Essential Oils and Bone Integrity

Performed by Bone Biology Group, Department of Clinical Research,
University of Bern, Switzerland (Muhlbauer, Lozano, Palacio, Reinli, Felix)

"Common Herbs, Essential Oils, and Monoterpenes Potently Modulate Bone Metabolism"

During our survey of herbs looking for activity on bone metabolism, we found that the dried leaves of sage strongly inhibit bone resorption. Therefore, we investigated several common herbs rich in essential oils (Sage, Rosemary, and Thyme) and essential oils extracted from these herbs and other plants (oils of Sage, Rosemary, Juniper, Pine, Dwarf Pine, Turpentine, and Eucalyptus) as well as their monoterpene components (thujone, eucalyptol, camphor, borneol, thymol, alpha-pinene, beta-pinene, bornylacetate as well as menthol) and found that they inhibit bone resorption when added to the food of rats. Pine oil, used as a representative essential oil, protects an osteoporosis model, the aged ovariectomized rat, from bone loss. The monoterpenes borneol, thymol, and camphor are directly inhibitory in the osteoclast [large cells responsible for the breakdown of bones] resorption pit assay. Nonpolar monoterpenes may require metabolism to be active in vitro, for example, cis-verbenol, a metabolite of alpha-pinene occurring in human urine, inhibits osteoclast activity in contrast to the parent compound. Within 30 min. borneol inhibits the formation of actin rings, a characteristic of resorbing osteoclasts indicating cell polarization. Both the in vitro and the in vivo effects of borneol are reversible. Our study demonstrates for the first time that essential oils and monoterpenes are efficient inhibitors of bone resorption in the rat.

fairness, it must be said that this approach did produce valuable insights. Even late in the twentieth century important discoveries were made. A few of the findings are mentioned here.

Anti-inflammative: Components in *Helichrysum italicum* have been shown to mediate their tissue protective and regenerative quality by effectively scavenging free radicals.[9]

Osteoporosis: Studies by Muhlbauer, Lozano, Palacio, Reinli, and Felix established common essential oils as unexpected and effective agents to prevent osteoporosis, the loss of bony tissue associated with low levels of estrogen.[10]

The Foundations of
Aromatherapy

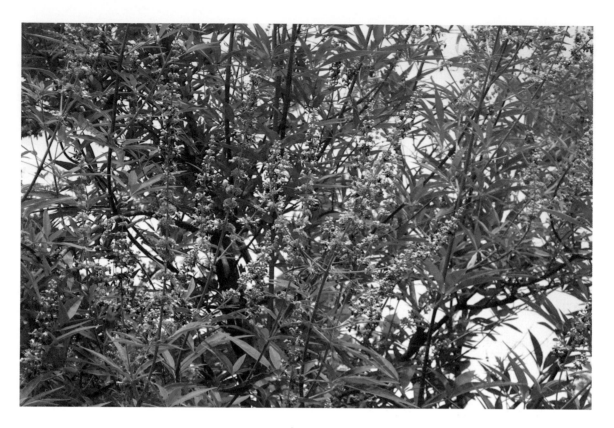

A very large specimen of *Vitex agnus castus* in the Ortobotanico of Padua: Vitex leaf essential oil is highly effective in re-equilibrating progesterone and estrogen, but its mechanism of action is not really understood.

PMS and menopausal complaints: *Vitex agnus castus* has been shown to be a singularly effective agent to re-equilibrate progesterone and estrogen levels and to have pronounced benefits for PMS and menopausal complaints.[11]

Hepatitis B and C: Long-term clinical studies by Dr. Anne-Marie Giraud-Robert have shown that various oils are effective in the treatment of hepatitis B and C, but no mechanisms have been proposed at this point (see chapter 15).[12]

Essential Oil Activity on the Cellular Plane

While conventional research led to many invaluable revelations about the healing properties of essential oils, many of the insights that have emerged more recently arise from innovative research taking place at the interface between chemistry and biology. To facilitate our discussion of these newly evolving concepts, we shall briefly present the understanding of cells, their makeup, and especially some of the relevant processes on the cellular level as they have been expressed in bio- and cellular chemistry in the last decades of the twentieth century.

The Fabric of Cells and Their Molecular Building Blocks

General Composition

- Water 80–85%
- Proteins 10–15%, functional components, enzymes, receptors, etc.
- Lipids 2–5%, phospholipids, membranes
- DNA 0.5%, genetic code
- RNA 0.5–1%, instrumental for protein synthesis
- Polysaccharides 0.1–1%, linked chains, backbone of the double helix
- Salt (Ions) 1.5%, vital for signaling

Amino Acids and Proteins

- The 10,000 different proteins of the human body are built of 20 amino acids.
- Essential amino acids are not produced by the human body.
- Amino acids have a carboxylic acid (acidic) and an amino group (alkaline).
- The presence of amino acids results in an amphoteric character.
- Carboxyl can bond with the amino group and form a peptide bond; by repeating this process amino acids can build chains.
- Long amino acids chains twist, fold, and rotate to form three-dimensional proteins.
- Hence proteins have the following types of structures:
  - *Primary
  - * Secondary (a-Helix, b-Sheet)
  - *Tertiary
  - * Quaternary

Phospholipids: The Skeleton of Biomembranes

- Glycerin is a C_3 molecule, where a hydroxyl (alcohol) group is attached to each carbon atom.
- As alcohols react with acids to form esters, both fatty acids and phosphoric acid react with glycerin to form a triester.
- Fatty acids are acidic because of their carboxyl group. Unsaturated fatty acids are a vital component of membrane phospholipids.
- Phosphoric acid is H_3PO_4.

- Phosphoric acid + glycerin = glycerin-3-phosphate (phosphoglycerin).
- Fatty acids can esterify with phosphoglycerin.
- The phosphate residue can continue to esterify (e.g., with cholin = trimethylethanolamin).

Sugar and Carbohydrates

- Sugars are polyalcohols with an aldehyde- or keto-group, called aldoses or ketoses.
- Sugars are named according to the number of C-atoms, trioses, tetroses, pentoses, hexoses, and so on.
- Sugars easily form rings: pyranoses, furanoses, in many different stereo-isomeric forms.
- Sugar can bond with sugar; the elimination of water creates a glucosidic bond.
- Several sugar molecules of the same or of different kind can form chains.

Nucleic Acids

DNA and RNA are nucleic acids: multiple molecules of different categories.

- Nucleic acids are natural polymers consisting of many nucleotide building blocks.
- Nucleotides consist of phosphoric acid, sugar (pentose), and base (pyrimidine and purine).
- DNA: the sugar is D-Deoxyribose; the bases can be thymine, cytosine, adenine, and guanine.
- RNA: the sugar is D-Ribose; the thymine base is replaced by uracil.

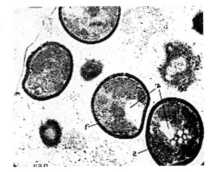

Induction of Liver Detoxification Enzymes

Many popular aromatherapy texts mention the ability of essential oils to stimulate detoxification. *The Practice of Aromatherapy* (the English translation of Jean Valnet's foundational text, *Aromathérapie,* published in 1964) states that Lemon oil is effective against liver stagnation. Today cellular and molecular biology let us understand why this is so! A large proportion of essential oil components induce so-called Phase I and Phase II liver detoxification enzymes. That this capacity was recognized by traditional healing systems specifically for Lemon oil is probably more a consequence of its ample availability and easy use than singular efficacy.

Liver detoxification is a two-tiered process. First the cytochrome P 450 enzymes (CYP), a large group of enzymes with a variety of functions, modify substances foreign to the body through oxidative degradation (breakdown of molecules as a consequence of oxidation). Just one of the subforms of CYP—CYP 3A4—metabolizes approximately 50 percent of all pharmaceuticals, while CYP 2D6 metabolizes approximately 30 percent and CYP 2C9 approximately 10 percent.

Once oxidation by Phase I enzymes has made foreign substances chemically more responsive, the Phase II enzymes add water-soluble "soft" molecules to the reaction products of the Phase I transformation. The end result is a composite molecule, which can be easily eliminated via the urinary tract.

SCIENTIFIC CONTEXT

Eliminating Alcohol from the Body

The intense way in which we depend on our liver detoxification enzymes in daily life is illustrated by the removal of alcohol, as in wine or cocktails.

The oxidation of alcohol (ethanol) is a culturally important enzymatic reaction. If the specific cytochrome enzyme 2E1 did not deploy rapidly after we start drinking a glass of wine, alcohol concentrations in the body would reach dangerous levels quickly. In this context it is interesting to note that not all xenobiotics induce Phase I enzymes. Some also inhibit their release, for instance the mix of essential oils and flavors in Coca-Cola. As Coca-Cola inhibits Phase I CYPs, alcohol is removed more slowly; as a result, rum and Coke is perceived as more intoxicating than an equivalent quantity of rum and, let's say, soda water!

$$CH_3.CH_2OH \longrightarrow \begin{array}{c} CH_3 \\ | \\ H-C-OH \\ | \\ OH \end{array} \longrightarrow CH_3.CHO + H_2O$$

The oxidation of ethanol by CYP 2E1

A general representation of the plasma membrane of a nerve cell. Phospholipids (the major structural lipids of most cellular membranes except the chloroplast) are oriented toward the inside and outside of the cell.

Glycolipids are exclusively oriented toward the outside. There is no general hypothesis for the almost total glycolization of surface proteins in nerve cells.

It appears obvious that galactose, though situated at the outside of the membrane, contributes directly (as well as by forming bonds with ligands) to vital information and control processes in the body. Galactose (a sugar similar to glucose), along with the phospholipids and cholesterol, is a fundamental and structural substance for cells, cell walls, and intracellular matrix.

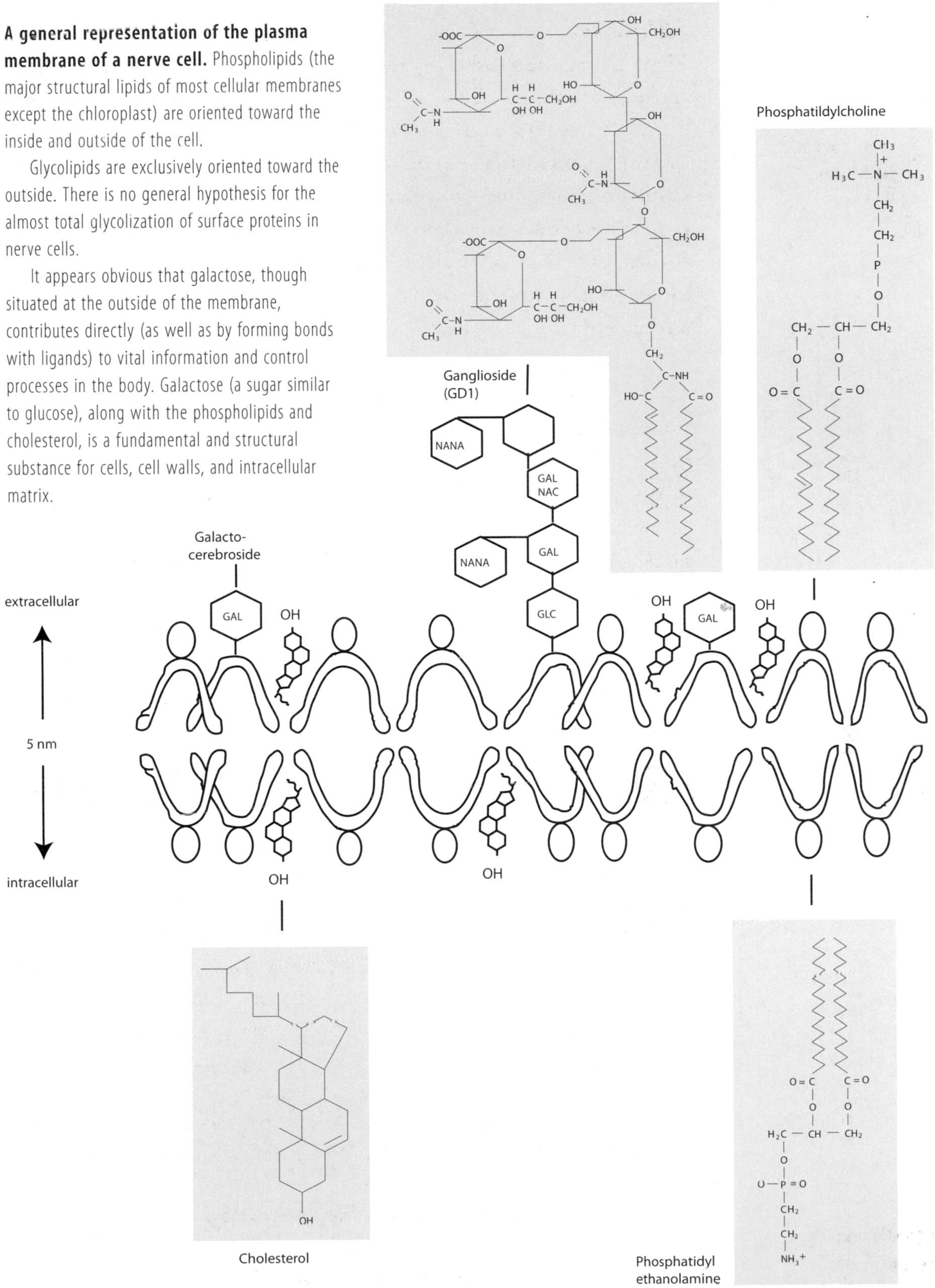

Phosphatildylcholine

Ganglioside (GD1)

NANA

GAL NAC

NANA

GAL

GLC

Galacto-cerebroside

GAL

extracellular

5 nm

intracellular

GAL

Cholesterol

Phosphatidyl ethanolamine

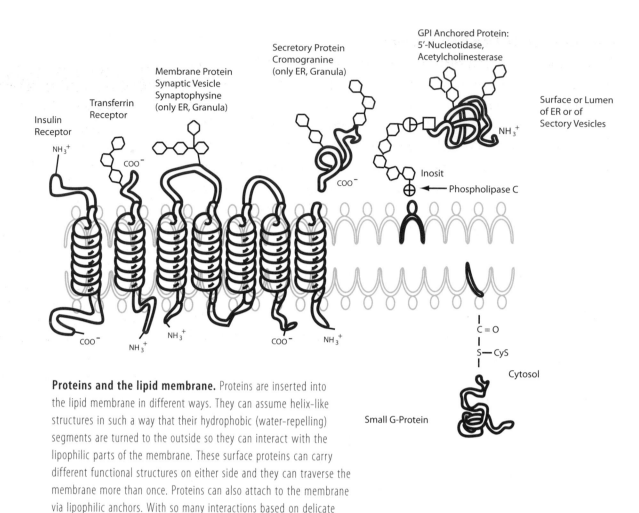

Proteins and the lipid membrane. Proteins are inserted into the lipid membrane in different ways. They can assume helix-like structures in such a way that their hydrophobic (water-repelling) segments are turned to the outside so they can interact with the lipophilic parts of the membrane. These surface proteins can carry different functional structures on either side and they can traverse the membrane more than once. Proteins can also attach to the membrane via lipophilic anchors. With so many interactions based on delicate balances of lipophilic and hydrophilic substances, it is no wonder that strongly lipophilic essential oils can cause any number of modifications to the cell membrane.

Inhibition of HMG CoA Reductase

HMG CoA reductase is a key enzyme in mammalian as well as plant life. It controls terpene, cholesterol, and ultimately sexual hormone synthesis.[13] Essential oils can inhibit this enzyme and thereby the synthesis of cholesterol, which in turn is relevant for the prevention or inhibition of carcinogenesis and tumor growth. The HMG CoA reductase enzyme in tumor cells is defective; it keeps producing much more cholesterol than normally needed, thereby sustaining the growth of the tumor. Research has demonstrated that the defective—permanently switched on—HMG CoA reductase of tumor cells is shut off (inhibited) by essential oils.

Interaction with Membrane Receptors

Surface proteins—receptors—in and on top of the cellular membrane are instrumental in regulating cellular processes. Receptors are membrane-bound or membrane-enclosed molecules that respond to mobile molecules, typically called ligands, with great specificity. Components of essential oils influence receptor activity in two ways. They can act as substrate for a receptor and thereby trigger whatever biological activity is induced by the specific receptor. Often these essential oil–receptor interactions result in a change in ion flow or electric potentials across the cell membrane and hence have antispasmodic or similar relaxing effects.

The second, indirect, way in which essential oils influence receptor activity is by modifying the expression and formation of the receptors. Studies performed on loggers in Sweden showed that their exposure to the terpenoids of the needle trees increased metabolic turnover as well as expression of surface proteins.[14]

Interaction with Nuclear Receptors

Receptors are the initial agents that transmit outside messages into the cell, which trigger biological responses. While the purpose and function of receptors present in the cellular membrane are relatively well understood, receptors sitting on the surface of the cell nucleus largely remain a scientific puzzle in evolutionary biology. Their function is not clear at this time. It is, however, obvious that the native substrates or ligands that interact with these receptors are either endogenous or from the natural world. An example is farnesene, present in many floral essential oils, which attaches directly to the farnesene receptor on the cell nucleus.[15]

Inflammation Mediators

Translation factors such as NF-kappa beta are key regulators of inflammatory and immune responses. They are essential for the transcription of multiple pro-inflammatory molecules. Sesquiterpene lactones, for instance, from Arnica herb or *Inula graveolens* or *Tanacetum annuum* essential oil, have been demonstrated to be effective against inflammatory processes by preventing activation of translation factors such as NF-kappa beta by different inflammation stimuli.[16]

Conclusion

Initial scientific knowledge about physiological effects of essential oils developed within the framework of the active ingredient concept. For most of the twentieth century the physiological effects of essential oils were explained as the consequence of a specific, physiologically active, component with a specific molecular structure. This rationale was congruent with the way single component drugs from aspirin to prozac could be understood. It became the accepted—and basically the only—way to understand physiological activity of natural substances.

Lemongrass and its main component citral serve as a good example. Since citral showed efficacy in some of the "crude" pharmacological models of the time, it was deemed the active ingredient. In the mind of the early twentieth-century chemist, Lemongrass oil had value because it contained citral. Two assumptions went into this way of thinking:

A. The active ingredient was responsible for the physiological effect of the oil.
B. The effect, that is, a spasmolytic effect, was the intrinsic property of the citral molecule.

While assumption A is slowly giving way (at least in aromatherapy circles) to the understanding that essential oils display healing properties as a consequence of all the substances present in an oil, assumption B—that healing properties are the intrinsic quality of a molecule—has survived mostly unchallenged. Prior to the most recent understanding, pharmacology considered it patently irrational to entertain the idea that the effect of a substance was not based in its molecular makeup. While the concept of molecular agency has allowed us to build an enormous body of knowledge about essential oils, it has also become a trap, as it has subjected essential oils and aromatherapy to the limitations of pharmacology and reductionist thought.

More recently the perspectives of organicism and evolutionary biology have come to remedy this. They provide rational explanations for phenomena too complex for a reductionist narrative. This development is of the highest significance for aromatherapy. To explore we shall proceed step by step.

TWO

THE BIOACTIVITY OF ESSENTIAL OILS

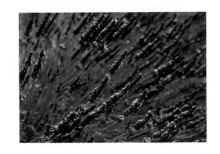

When he took what had come to be his usual solitary evening stroll along the terrace or beside the lotus pool, he felt an extraordinary sense of mental and physical settlement.

JAMES HILTON, *LOST HORIZON*

In line with conventional medical research, the explanation of essential oil efficacy was focused for the longest time on the pharmacology of isolated chemical components. As our culture prizes medical and drug science almost above everything else, we began to overlook that essential oils are part and parcel of living nature.

Ignoring the biological nature of essential oils has inhibited aromatherapy. It led to the tacit assumption that there is a similarity in the therapeutic use of essential oils and conventional drugs. As a result, the language used for the prescription and application of essential oils generally resembles that of conventional medicines.

But equating essential oils with man-made drugs, simply because we can give chemical formulas for the constituents of both, leads to fundamentally incorrect conclusions. Man-made drugs are produced in factories, reflecting at best human ingenuity and at worst Enron-style exploitation. They often are a synthesis of our culture of war with the latest achievement of corporate science. Reflecting our culture, they are intended to fight pathogens, disease, germs, cancer, infections, and, lately, those aspects of our lifestyles that are somehow deemed undesirable.

To overcome those limitations, aromatherapy has to stop mimicking drug science and give renewed recognition to the fact that essential

SCIENTIFIC CONTEXT

Ernst Mayr

Ernst Mayr is professor emeritus of zoology at Harvard University. He ranks among the most eminent biologists of the twentieth century and has given evolutionary biology many important impulses. He is author and editor of many books in his field. In 1997 he published *This is Biology*, an eloquent and immensely readable introduction to the character and development of biological thinking and the science of life itself.

Exploring Transcultural Constants

Angelica Root, German and Roman Chamomile, Hops, and Lovage Root or Yarrow are typical essential oils from the moderate climates of central Europe. These plants and their essential oils are more or less transcultural constants. Where there is beer, there is Hops. Lovage Root apparently has a composition practically identical to the Chinese staple Dong Quai. *Angelica archangelica* is historically credited with many healing properties. Interestingly the Chinese description given by Taoist Master Jeffrey Yuen addresses the most easily utilized quality of the essential oil. It supports the spleen in separating the indigestible from the nutritious and quickly restores weight to those who are asthenic or underweight. In addition authentic Angelica root, and to a lesser degree seed oils, delight with the most pronounced musk note.

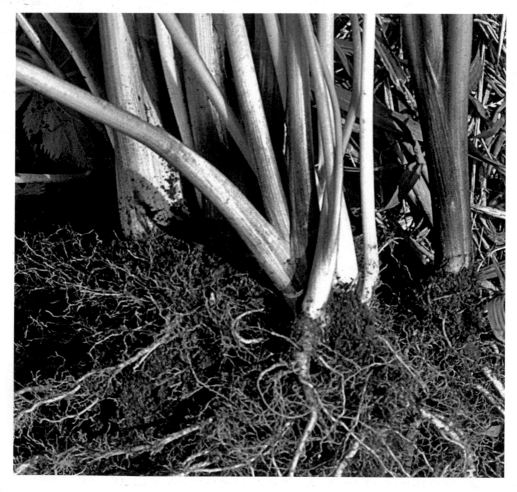

Angelica archangelica roots

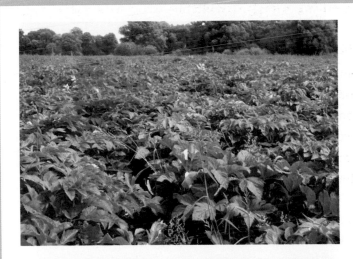

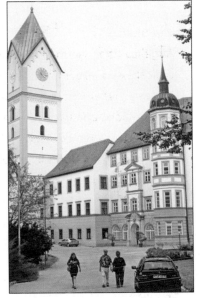

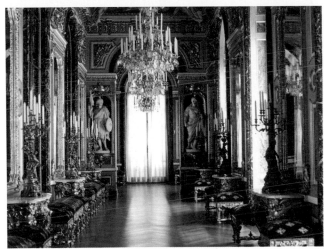

Plants that thrive in moderate climates, such as Angelica, German Chamomile, and Lovage, do well in Bavaria, which surprises the visitor with its duality of strong agricultural tradition and the splendor of an absolutist past.

Above left: Angelica cultivation
Above right: Kloster Scheyern
Left: Herrenchiemsee

oils arise from nature. Their activity is shaped by the ambient ways of the plant world. Essential oils do not act as weapons but as agents of interaction. They are a key ingredient of life itself, strengthening its fabric and preconditions.

The Quantum Leap: Organicism

As outlined in chapter 1, for most of the twentieth century, the physiological effects of an essential oil were explained by making reference to the molecular structure of an active ingredient. This language reflects the core belief that everything, including living organisms, can be

The Bioactivity of
Essential Oils

SCIENTIFIC CONTEXT

Organicism—
Organization of Living
Organisms

Social Levels:
Societies
Social Groups

Biological Levels:
Individuals
Supersystems (e.g., central nervous
system)
Organs (e.g., hypothalamus)
Cells (e.g., neurons)

Chemical Levels:
Organelles (e.g., ribosomes)
Molecules (e.g., DNA)

Physical Levels:
Atoms (e.g., Ca)
Subatomic particles

explained by the laws of chemistry and physics. The corresponding philosophical position was called *physicalism* in the early twentieth century. Physicalism is the thesis that the nature of the universe and everything in it conforms to the condition of being physical. Physicalists don't deny that the world might contain phenomena that at first glance don't seem physical—phenomena of a biological, psychological, moral, or social nature. But they insist nevertheless that ultimately such items are either physical or caused by the physical. *Vitalism,* on the other hand, held that living organisms are fundamentally different from nonliving entities because they contain some nonphysical element or are governed by different principles than are inanimate things. Its proponents believed that there was something akin to a life force, which was not accessible with the laws of physics or chemistry. The scientific battles between the two camps could not be settled by even more physics. Instead they were resolved by modern biology and the emergence of a new concept: *organicism.*

Organicism holds that within the organizational hierarchy of living organisms (emergent) properties arise at each level of organization. These properties cannot be predicted by even the most detailed knowledge (i.e., physical and molecular) of a lower level of organization. This has direct consequences for the study of aromatherapy, for essential oils are produced by the whole plant organism and, in their constantly varying composition, reflect the interaction of the plant with its environment. They are thus the vehicle for much of the plant's communication with and relation to the outside world.

Even the slightest grasp of the utter complexity of life makes it obvious that the plant organism has vested certain properties in essential oils, which arise at that very refined level of interaction between plants and other plants as well as between plants and mammals. A semi-humorous and semi-serious example may illustrate this: looking at the molecule methyl chavicol, the main component of basil oil, does not explain why pesto is made with basil and not with tarragon, which has the same main component. It also does not explain why pesto is a staple of the Mediterranean cuisine and not of Dutch cooking.

Grasping that properties can in fact emerge at the level of a whole organism unmasks the mantra-like recitation of chemical components as a wildly overrated exercise when it comes to explaining the full range of essential oil properties. While scientists were aware that secondary

E. O. Wilson

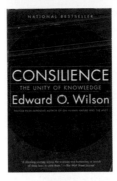

E. O. Wilson has influenced public consciousness in the United States and globally in ways hard to overestimate. In *The Diversity of Life* he has advocated an understanding of the value of diversity and the risks humanity runs if diversity is destroyed. In *Consilience* Wilson argues for a confluence of all science on the basis of physics and chemistry.

Wendell Berry

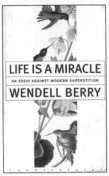

Wendell Berry responded to Wilson's *Consilience* with an essay against modern superstition. For Berry the idea that life could be explained only through molecules and physics is plain laughable. The argument between Wilson and Berry is a most captivating modern version of the physicalist/vitalist debate, where both protagonists are most convincing and eloquent.

---

plant metabolites play many interesting roles, such as signaling from plant to insects, the full scope of their activities and interactions with life in general was missed. A fundamental change in paradigm is only happening now.

Secondary Plant Metabolites: Physiologically Active by Design

Secondary metabolites are made by the plant even though they are not necessary for its immediate survival or its day-to-day economy. They do not participate in the metabolic processes of deriving energy from nutrition or the propagation of the species. They do, however, contribute to the mid- and long-term success of the plant by ensuring its survival vis-à-vis competing organisms and by improving its odds for reproduction. This is a rather tall order, considering the limitations of plant life. Plants do not have an immune system, but they need to resist the challenges of bacteria, fungi, and viruses. They need to defend against herbivores and

The Bioactivity of
Essential Oils

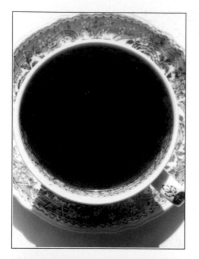

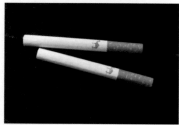

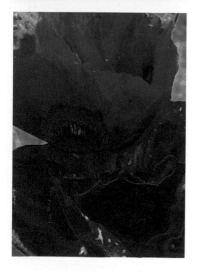

Secondary metabolites

attract pollinators. In short, they face complex requirements in relating to the world around them.

Since plants do not speak or move, the need to relate to other plants and animals was answered by developing molecules that trigger physiological responses in other organisms, in this context referred to as "target organisms." These molecules, the secondary metabolites, influence the behavior of a target organism in the interest of the plant! They defend or attract, but they also produce other specific interactions.

Secondary metabolites achieve this by connecting not with one but with a variety of physiological processes of the target organism. The three main molecular targets modified by plant secondary metabolites are:

- Proteins
- DNA and RNA
- Biological membranes (or biomembranes)

To reach this degree of efficiency, secondary plant metabolites underwent intense molecular modeling over the long time periods of biological evolution and, because of this, reflect the genius of life itself. The intricate and intense ways in which secondary metabolites are an integral part of the whole symphony of life make their actions fundamentally different from those of synthetic medicines.

From the perspective of aromatherapy there is one more consideration. The plant uses its innate biochemical pathways to generate a broad structural diversity of secondary metabolites, including essential oil components, flavonoids, alkaloids, saponins, and pigments. Most of those are polar (better soluble in water than the nonpolar essential oil components) and of higher molecular weight. They remain within the plant organism and display their effect once a herbivore or microorganism tries to feed on the plant. In contrast terpenoids and phenylpropanoids are lipophilic and volatile (easily evaporated). They are among the plant's main means to communicate with other organisms over a distance.

Defensive Strategies and Molecular Targets

Plants need to be able to defend against a wide variety of attackers. This requires a broad spectrum of activity, because a substance that might

Plant Evolution, a Summary

The Beginning

- Earth is 4.5 billion years old.
- Fossils are 3.5 billion years old.
- The first cells consisted of carbon, oxygen, hydrogen, and nitrogen.
- 98% of all living organisms are composed of these elements.

Photosynthesis Changed Earth's Atmosphere

- Self-sustaining (autotrophic) organisms began to split water (H_2O), utilizing the hydrogen and releasing the oxygen (O_2) into the atmosphere.
- As the O_2 in the atmosphere converted to O_3, the O_3 became sufficient to absorb UV light.
- Organisms protected from UV by the ozone layer began to develop 450 million years ago.
- The increased availability of O_2—originally toxic to the anaerobic organisms—was turned into a virtue. Respiration developed.

Humans Need Plants

- Chlorophyll enables photosynthesis.
- Photosynthesis transforms light energy into chemical energy usable by living organisms.
- Photosynthesis is the connection between animate and inanimate nature: it is the means by which self-sustaining or self-nourishing (autotrophic) cell-like structures generate organic molecules from simple inorganic molecules.
- Plants are autotrophic; they can generate the carbohydrates they need from the CO_2 in the air.
- Humans are heterotrophic, dependent upon nourishment by intake and digestion of organic matter.
- Human survival is completely dependent on plants.

Prokaryotes and Eukaryotes

There are two categories of cells: prokaryotes and eukaryotes. Before oxygen accumulated in the atmosphere there were only prokaryotic cells (bacteria and blue green algae, characterized by a simple naked chromosome). As oxygen became abundant eukaryotic cells (with chromosomes in a nucleus, separated from the cytoplasm by membranes) arose.

Prokaryotes: single-celled organisms without a nucleus

- Prokaryotic cell DNA is not attached or contained in a nucleus.
- Prokaryotic cell size ranges from 0.1 to 1 micrometer (1 micrometer equals $1/1{,}000$ of a millimeter.
- Prokaryotic cells have no internal compartments or cytoskeleton.

Eukaryotes: cells with compartments or organelles

Organelles are specific areas of the cell, housing specific physiological processes separated by enclosing biological membranes or biomembranes. They include:

- Nucleus (the major organelle, separating the chromosomes from the cytoplasm)
- Mitochondria (highly variable structures containing many enzymes)
- Vacuole (large vesicles)
- Plastids (often containing elaborate internal membrane systems, the best-known representative being the chloroplast that houses photosynthesis)
- Golgi apparatus (an intracellular stack of vesicles in which packaging of secreted proteins takes place)
- Endoplasmatic reticulum (membrane system that branches out through the cytoplasm of the cell)

The Secret Life of Plants was published in 1973 and became an instant cult classic. It was far ahead of its time in the recognition of many of the sensitivities and capabilities of plants, which almost seemed absurd to the scientific orthodoxy of the time.

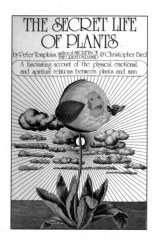

keep a caterpillar away might be some beetle's fancy. To answer this need plants have adopted a strategy that is universally effective: they have developed secondary metabolites that modify functional proteins (essentially receptors and enzymes) in the target organism, thereby modifying the processes these proteins perform. This can be a highly effective deterrent, since proteins performing the functions of receptors and enzymes are the main players in practically all cellular processes. Upsetting the functioning of the enzymatic processes performed by these proteins can significantly deter an attacker!

Secondary metabolites perform their defensive tasks in two principal ways. Some interact selectively with specific receptors, but a majority operate in nonselective ways.

Selective Binding to Proteins

A fair number of secondary metabolites have evolved that bind to specific surface proteins or neuroreceptors. This type of specific binding of secondary metabolites is found mostly among plant alkaloids. In the realm of essential oils some sesquiterpenes bind to specific receptors.[1]

Secondary plant metabolites with selective activity are generally well understood. Selective activity is found in those secondary metabolites that feature a high degree of structural similarity to (endogenous) mammalian hormones and neurotransmitters (substances found in chemical synapses, the connections between two excitable cells, crucial for transduction of electric signals). In other words, plants have managed to model secondary metabolites to closely resemble neurotransmitters such as acetylcholine, serotonin, noradrenalin, dopamine, GABA, and histamine, and hormones like endorphins. This type of secondary metabolite can attach to the same receptors as the endogenous messenger molecules.

In cases like those of heart glycosides, salicylic derivatives from the willow tree, or quinine from the bark of the cinchona tree, selective activity of the respective secondary metabolites has been demonstrated by experimental pharmacology. Consequently these plant products have been integrated into the arsenal of conventional medicine.

In his *Diversity of Life,* biologist E. O. Wilson points out that few of us are aware of how much we already depend on wild organisms for medicine.

Aspirin, the most widely used pharmaceutical in the world, was derived from salicylic acid discovered in meadowsweet (*Filipendula ulmaria*) and later combined with acetic acid to create acetylsalicylic acid, the more effective painkiller. In the United States a quarter of all prescriptions dispensed by pharmacies are substances extracted from plants. Another 13 percent come from microorganisms and 3 percent more from animals, for a total of over 40 percent that are organism-derived. Yet these materials are only a tiny fraction of the multitude available. Fewer than 3 percent of the flowering plants of the world, about 5,000 of the 220,000 species, have been examined for alkaloids, and then in limited and haphazard fashion. The anticancer potency of the rosy periwinkle was discovered by the merest chance, because the species happened to be widely planted and under investigation for its reputed effectiveness as an antidiuretic.

The scientific and folkloric record is strewn with additional examples of plants and animals valued in folk medicine but still unaddressed in biomedical research. The Neem tree (*Azadirachta indica*), a relative of mahogany, is a native of tropical Asia virtually unknown in the developed world. The people of India, according to a recent report of the U.S. National Research Council, treasure the species. "For centuries, millions have cleaned their teeth with neem twigs, smeared skin disorders with neem-leaf juice, taken neem tea as a tonic, and placed neem leaves in their beds, book, grain bins, cupboards, and closets to keep away troublesome bugs. The tree has relieved so many different pains, fevers, infections, and other complaints that it has been called the 'village pharmacy.' To those millions in India neem has miraculous powers, and now scientists around the world are beginning to think they may be right."

One should never dismiss the reports of such powers as superstition or legend. Organisms are superb chemists. In a sense they are collectively better than all the world's chemists at synthesizing organic molecules of practical use. Through millions of generations each kind of plant, animal, and microorganism has experimented with chemical substances to meet its special needs. Each species has experienced astronomical numbers of mutations and genetic recombinations affecting its biochemical machinery. The experimental products thus produced have been tested by the unyielding forces of natural selection, one generation at a time. The special class of

The Bioactivity of Essential Oils

chemicals in which the species became a wizard is precisely determined by the niche it occupies.[2]

While their actions are well understood, the similarity between the molecular structures of human hormones and neurotransmitters and the almost picture-perfect imitations produced by plants is still surprising. How is it possible that a plant can produce molecules that are almost mirrors of substances in humans or other mammals? The answer is seldom discussed: metabolism in plants and mammals is very similar and partly even identical. Proteins, enzymes, and the general biochemical machinery (the primary metabolism) of all life has an extremely high degree of uniformity. All molecules of life arise from the same ancestral biochemical machinery of prokaryotic cells. And all multicell organisms share the biochemistry of eukaryotic cells, identical biological assembly lines often producing very similar and even identical molecules. Biochemical diversity arises with the products of the secondary metabolism.

Nonselective Binding to Proteins

The disturbance of a protein's three-dimensional structure, or its *conformation*, appears to be a major strategy of plants when selecting molecules for defense. In the course of evolution plants have learned, by means of their secondary metabolites, to impair or alter the proper functioning of proteins in the target organism by disturbing their conformation. In the case of an enzyme this will, subtly or strongly, change the activity of the enzyme.

Secondary metabolites that disturb protein conformation generally act nonselectively: they interact with structural features found in all or almost all proteins. Two main strategies are followed to modify protein conformation. One is to form covalent chemical bonds (bonds between two atoms mediated by a pair of electrons) with particular structural elements of proteins (such as NH_2 terminals or SH groups). The other is by so-called weak interactions (such as when lipophilic terpene molecules insert themselves into the lipophilic segments of a protein and thereby change its conformation). These strategies affect all proteins that present the requisite molecular targets, regardless of their specific function.

Certain plant molecules have structural elements that readily undergo covalent binding to proteins (such as at the aforementioned

Fine-Tuning of Secondary Metabolites

Given the drastic shift in perception introduced by evolutionary biology, some reflection about the process of evolution seems in order. In the Darwinian view of evolution there is no purpose. Instead, those plants that happened to produce a selection of secondary metabolites that favored their survival were successful. They reproduced more successfully than others, and in doing so, they reproduced the biochemical machinery that generated that successful set of secondary metabolites.

Conversely, those plants whose secondary metabolites did not increase their chances of survival—such as by not fending off herbivores effectively—did not reproduce as successfully or died out. With them vanished the lesser-suited combination of secondary metabolites. Only the most fine-tuned composition of secondary metabolites is able to ensure continued success of a given plant species.

NH$_2$ or SH sites). As the overall chemical structure of the protein changes through the addition (binding) of the additional molecule, so does its conformation. Essential oil molecules that can react in this way and significantly distort protein conformation by nonselective binding are, for instance, terpene aldehydes as found in Melissa or Lemongrass.

Protein conformation can also be modified when terpenes of an essential oil interact with the lipophilic areas of a protein. The small lipophilic terpenes can insert themselves into lipophilic areas of a protein and thereby change its conformation. Such interactions are called weak interactions because no actual chemical bonds are formed.

Molecular Target: DNA, RNA, and Gene Expression

Many plants contain secondary metabolites that can cause mutations and malformations (by alkylating DNA bases, by intercalating or inserting themselves between base pairs of DNA, or by oxidizing DNA). These interactions are powerful means for plants to defend against microbes and even herbivores, if not immediately, certainly in the long run. A large share of this activity is mediated by so-called epoxides (molecules with a structural element where two carbons and one oxygen form a ring), which tend to react with many biological substrates, DNA among them. Epoxides are generally not found in essential oils and are generally avoided in phytotherapy.

Secondary metabolites have yet another way to modify, not necessarily DNA itself, but gene expression. Humans have about twenty-five thousand genes, which are expressed in different cells and organs in a differential fashion. Specific transcription factors (another type of functional protein) are present, which regulate gene expression. The covalent and noncovalent modifications of proteins described above also affect transcription factors. Preliminary experiments show that mixtures of secondary metabolites as they occur in plants can trigger the expression of several hundred genes, which are relevant in different pathways.

Molecular Target: Cell Membrane

The cell membrane separates the reaction space of the cell from the surrounding environment. Without cell membranes, there would not have been any evolution of higher life-forms. Nerve and tissue cells are surrounded by a double lipid layer membrane 5 nanometers wide. Most water-soluble molecules cannot penetrate the membrane, only nonpolar

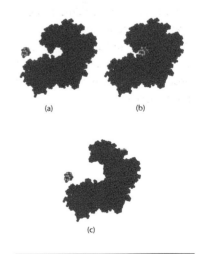
The Bioactivity of
Essential Oils

or very small molecules like O_2, CO_2, or water can permeate the membrane uninhibited. The necessary exchanges of amino acids, sugars, and signaling are performed by proteins integrated into the membrane.

One of the most outstanding qualities of nerve and sensory cells is their ability to generate and conduct electric signals. This is the result of the membranes' ability to separate charges and the ability of specific membrane proteins (ion pumps) to affect controlled changes in conductivity. Many of the effects of essential oil molecules are a consequence of their ability to modify this electric signaling. They do so by modifying membrane function two ways:

1. They can either insert themselves into the lipid membrane, creating hydrophobic interactions with the lipophilic chains of the phospholipids or cholesterol. In this fashion the terpenes in essential oils change membrane fluidity or permeability and ultimately structure and functionality.
2. Essential oil molecules can change membrane function by attaching to the lipophilic areas of membrane proteins, that is,

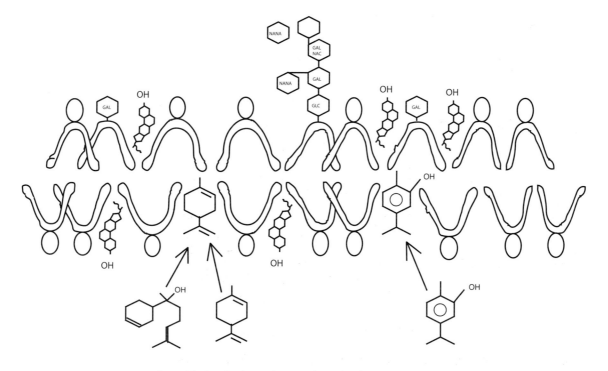

Essential oil molecules easily insert themselves between the lipophilic elements of the phospholipid membrane. By altering the structure of the membrane, the functionality of the receptors and ion channels embedded in the membrane is affected.

receptor proteins. As terpenoids form hydrophobic interactions with those segments of the receptor, which are themselves lodged in the membrane, they modify its conformation (its three-dimensional structure) and hence functionality. A well-known example for this is the interference of terpenoids with the ion channels in nerve cell membranes, modifying neuromuscular activity to relieve spasms at smooth intestinal muscle cells. Interference of high concentrations of terpenoids with membranes also mediates their narcotic and anesthetic effects.

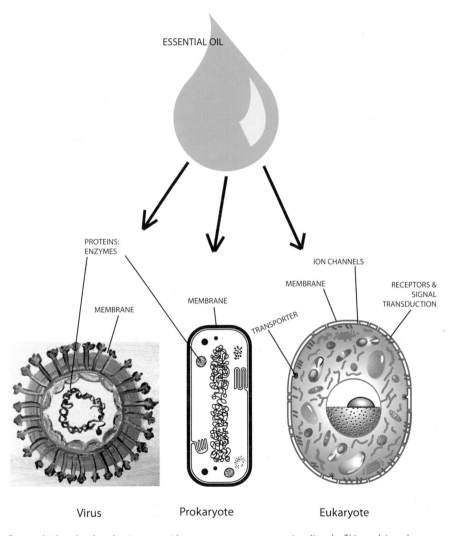

ESSENTIAL OIL

PROTEINS:
ENZYMES

MEMBRANE

MEMBRANE

TRANSPORTER

ION CHANNELS

MEMBRANE

RECEPTORS &
SIGNAL
TRANSDUCTION

Virus   Prokaryote   Eukaryote

Essential oil molecules also interact with receptor or enzyme proteins directly. This explains why essential oils have a much broader spectrum of action than, for instance, conventional antibiotic drugs. Antibiotics generally inhibit specific processes in the formation of the cell membrane of prokaryotic cells. They are much less effective vis-à-vis eukaryotic cells and ineffective against viruses.

The Bioactivity of
Essential Oils

Summation of Physiological Activity of Secondary Plant Metabolites

To recap, secondary plant metabolites utilize a variety of strategies to connect with molecular targets:

- Selective interaction with specific molecular targets such as neuro- or hormone receptors
- Disturbance of the three-dimensional structure of proteins
- Covalent bonding to DNA and RNA, modifying gene expression
- Changing membrane permeability and the function of membrane proteins

Only the first mechanism—the interaction of a secondary metabolite with an active site of a protein—is selective and specific. Such interactions are very powerful, but their disadvantage is that they are generally restricted to a small number of enemies who have the specific target.

Molecules that disturb the conformation of proteins, the structure of DNA and RNA, or the fluidity of membranes are obviously nonselective. Such molecules interact with many different targets. Although nonspecific, these interactions are very effective, because they disturb molecular targets in whatever enemy attacks the plant.

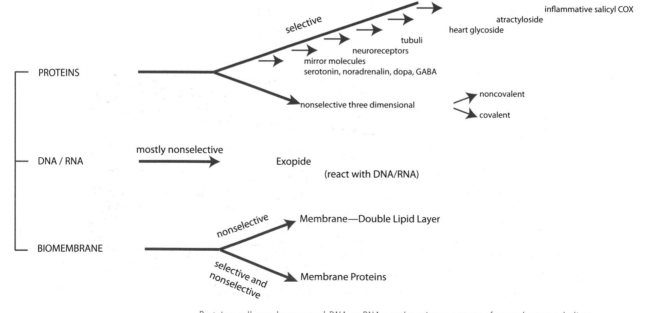

Proteins, cell membranes, and DNA or RNA are the primary targets of secondary metabolites. Selective interactions occur when secondary metabolites attach to specific receptor proteins. A much larger number of nonselective interactions occur through covalent or noncovalent interactions with structural elements of proteins.

Plant Expression

Identical Molecules Convey Different Messages:
Eucalyptus and Ravintsara

Different plant species can apparently package very different physiological messages by at least partially using identical chemical components. A good example of this is provided by *Eucalyptus radiata* and *Cinnamomum camphora* (Ravintsara).

Chemical analysis reveals both essential oils to be cineole-rich compositions with a preponderance of standard terpene hydrocarbons and terpene alcohols. Nonetheless, everyone working with these oils knows their distinctly different properties. One example is the tonifying effect Ravintsara has on the nervous system, which is not observed in the *Eucalyptus radiata*. This difference is not obvious from the chemical composition of both oils.

The *Cinnamomum camphora* tree is native to Taiwan, southern Japan, southeast China, and Indochina. It is a chemical chameleon from which different essential oils are derived. The oil called Ravintsara represents a cineole type. *Ho* is the vernacular name for its linalool type produced in Vietnam. Additionally, botanists distinguish a nerolidol, a safrole, and a borneol type. The name-giving substance, camphor, was historically derived by distilling the wood.

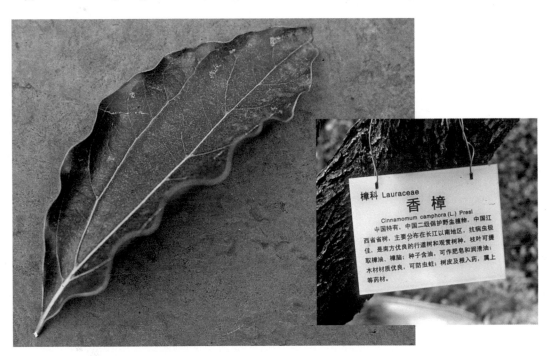

Ravintsara (*Cinnamomum camphora*) is effectively used topically. Because of its mild nature and tonifying character, it also lends itself to internal use.

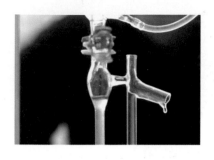

THREE

FROM BIOLOGY TO AROMATHERAPY

Biology comprises all disciplines dedicated to the exploration of living organisms.

ERNST MAYR

In chapter 2 we explored how plants developed substances directed at the world around them. In this chapter we shall explore how mammals answered and how the back and forth of evolution creates a dense web of interactions, the fabric of life! And we shall see the implications of that for the practice of plant medicine.

The Evolution of Liver Detoxification Enzymes

Understanding how liver detoxification enzymes—and with them the capacity to remove substances foreign to the body—arose is instructive. It illustrates why benefits from plant secondary metabolites are so diverse and how we derive benefits we may not even recognize.

As humans spread out over planet Earth, they were continuously forced to adapt to new and unfamiliar environments and as a consequence to new and unfamiliar food. Plants contain digestible nutrients such as proteins, carbohydrates, fats, and oils, as well as indigestible secondary metabolites (alkaloids, flavonoids, phenylpropanes, and terpenes—essential oils—among many others). Originally these secondary metabolites were more or less toxic to the mammalian organism. Over time the mammals adjusted by developing an enzymatic machinery capable of processing these indigestible components, so they could

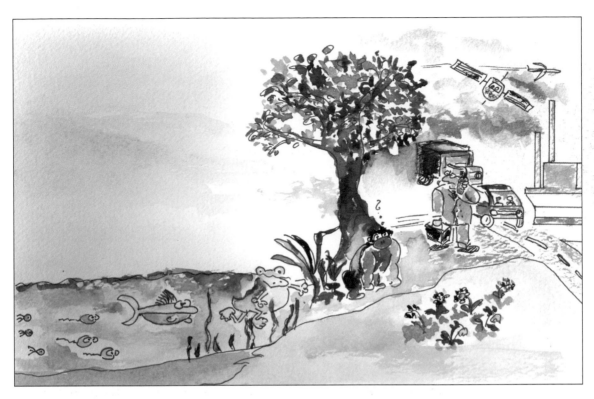

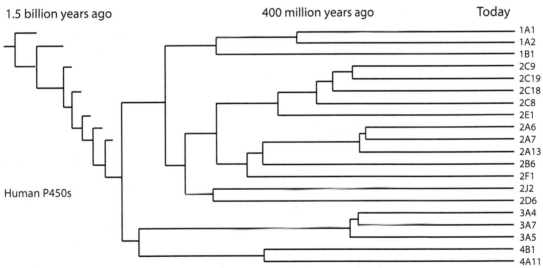

1.5 billion years ago   400 million years ago   Today

1A1
1A2
1B1
2C9
2C19
2C18
2C8
2E1
2A6
2A7
2A13
2B6
2F1
2J2
2D6
3A4
3A7
3A5
4B1
4A11

Human P450s

Evolution of cytochrome P450 (Phase I) liver detoxification enzymes
(original watercolor by Monika Haas)

safely be eliminated. To emphasize the point: essential oils are among the native agents responsible for the development of the liver detoxification enzymes and especially for those with the ability to remove lipophilic xenobiotics (lipophilic substances foreign to the body). Thus the

To accomplish the degradation of foreign molecules, Phase I enzymes metabolize substrates into reactive intermediates. Phase II enzymes (UDP glucuronosyl transferases, glutathione S-transferases, and N-acetyl transferases) then bind these intermediates to water-soluble molecules, completing the detoxification cycle. P450 induction usually enhances detoxification; thus, under most conditions, induction is a protective mechanism. Induction is likely to be advantageous in the evolution of species, allowing enhanced detoxification following exposure to xenobiotics.

system of cytochrome P450 enzymes (CYP)—as the various Phase I liver detoxification enzymes are also called—developed to its current state.[1]

CYPs are usually described as "liver detoxification systems" or "chemical defense against xenobiotic compounds of our environment." Today "xenobiotic compounds of our environment" include drugs and environmental pollutants. Once a modest set of only a few cytochromes, it is now an assortment of at least twenty commonly employed cytochromes with genes in our DNA coding for about forty more, which apparently are not utilized. It is clear that CYPs first evolved to detoxify dietary and endogenous products. The fact that they also detoxify drugs and pollutants proves the success of the "nonselective" strategy.

Secondary Metabolites: Dynamic Removal of Toxins

The development of the enzymes that now are part and parcel of our metabolic makeup was triggered by our coexistence and coevolution with the plant world and its secondary metabolites. This alone suggests that interacting with plants or plant products is vital to the healthy functioning of our metabolism. It also suggests that living on a diet of industrial foods, which were not part of the diet of our ancestors, may lead to the accumulation of toxins, as we do not have the necessary enzymes to remove the foreign non-nutrients inherent in such a diet.

The fact that we have enzymes in place that have specifically evolved to remove essential oils, formerly perceived by our systems as xenobiotics, explains why real toxicity among essential oil components is observed only in very few and easily identifiable instances.

Another aspect of liver detoxification has the highest impact for aromatherapy: not only do essential oils trigger their own biotransformation (chemical modification by an organism, typically by enzymes), but the process is also highly dynamic. Whenever the Phase I and II processes are activated by essential oils, much more enzyme than what would be needed to remove the original quantity of essential oil is produced. As a result previously accumulated toxins present in the liver are eliminated along with the essential oil molecules.

Resistance

It is well known that bacterial pathogens develop resistance to conventional antibiotics, often in the course of only a few years. This is a consequence of the narrow focus of antibiotics. They are generally highly selective, inhibiting a single mechanism in the formation or metabolism of the pathogen. When one microorganism has changed just enough to survive the antibiotic, it will replicate freely.

Essential oil components are fundamentally different. Their non-selective activity makes it practically impossible for microorganisms to develop resistance. Microorganisms may be able to resist the attack on one of their targets, but this leaves all the other targets of the essential oil still vulnerable.

In addition some targets are so central and important to the existence of the microorganism, such as respiration, that it cannot simply abandon them by a slight mutation. There is, for instance, no way in which a microorganism could counteract an attack on its membrane by lipophilic essential oils. The microorganism simply needs its membrane!

Limonene: The Complex Portfolio of Simple Molecules

Biological evolution, for the most part, did not produce secondary metabolites with very specific activity but rather components that can interact with multiple physiological systems. The simple limonene molecule, a major constituent of many Citrus and other oils, is a perfect example. Evolution has produced many substances like limonene, which support life by carrying the plant's message influencing the enzymatic machinery of the target organism. This is how a large number of apparently unrelated types of physiological activities arise, such as removing carcinogens, inhibiting tumor growth, and treating herpes lesions.

Limonene slightly inhibits Phase I liver detoxification enzymes, simultaneously inducing Phase II enzymes. The net result is that the production of potentially toxic or even carcinogenic intermediates, which sometimes occurs in the Phase I process, is slowed and the accelerated Phase II process removes them instantly. Under the influence of limonene, potential carcinogens cannot linger. This same limonene molecule selectively inhibits reproduction of tumor cells via the inhibition of HMG CoA reductase. These three effects—and most likely many additional ones—occur concurrently whenever we eat citrus fruits or use Lemon or Orange oil. These processes illustrate how complexity arises, ultimately giving natural plant extracts their unrivaled spectrum

Under some circumstances (like imbalance between Phase I and II enzymes after induction) it is possible that oxidation by cytochrome P450s leads to toxic, carcinogenic, mutagenic (causing an increased rate of mutation), or cytotoxic intermediate products. In this case toxicity depends upon balance between Phase I and II enzymes. If Phase II enzymes are depleted (for instance, as GSH is in alcoholics), these intermediates can linger and react with macromolecules such as DNA. However, if sufficient Phase II enzymes are available, the harmful intermediates are quickly processed and removed.

From Biology to Aromatherapy

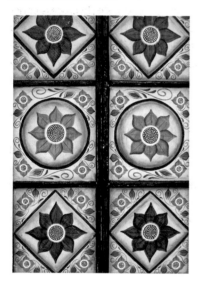

of activity. The different properties of limonene only appear unrelated because of our cultural—and economic—bias to seek cures for cancer separate from those for heart disease and also separate from limonene's influence on liver enzymes. The predilection for specific cures maximizes economic activity but clouds the awareness of health.

Multicomponent and Multitarget

Thus, important new impulses for aromatherapy are coming from evolutionary and cellular biology as they emphasize the hitherto barely recognized therapeutic relevance of multitarget strategies and the resulting nonselective effects of essential oils, which, contrary to the well-understood selective effects, have been all but ignored. Understanding the vast potential of the nonselective activity of essential oils opens up new treatment options for degenerative, autoimmune, and civilization diseases.

We have seen that plants developed secondary metabolites that can interact with the broadest variety of molecular targets. But plants did not stop there; they further refined their defensive capacity to match the diversity of the attackers. They apparently did not develop single substances, with one or two defensive capabilities, but complex mixtures of secondary metabolites, in which each component contributes multiple defensive capabilities. These mixtures simultaneously interfere with a large number of molecular targets in animals and in prokaryotic (bacteria) cells.

In "Evolutionary Advantage and Molecular Modes of Action of Multi-Component Mixtures in Phytomedicine," Michael Wink advocates the use of secondary metabolites in medicine and summarizes the areas in which the described activities are of the greatest therapeutic value:

> Plants use complex mixtures of secondary compounds of different structural classes to protect themselves against herbivores, bacteria, fungi and viruses. Because these secondary metabolites are not molecules with random structures, but active metabolites, which have been selected in the course of evolution, we can use them in medicine. Secondary metabolites, which plants use to defend against bacteria fungi or viruses, can be used in almost the same way in medicine to treat microbial or viral infections.[2]

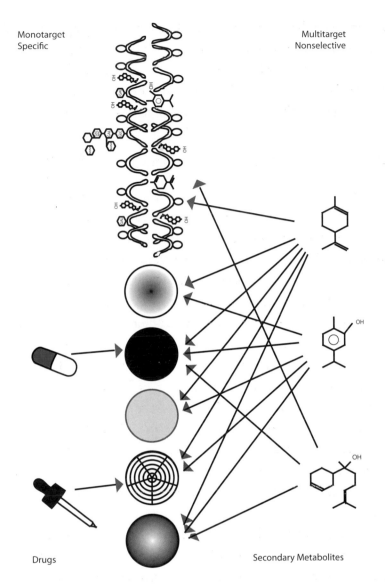

Monotarget
Specific

Multitarget
Nonselective

Drugs

Secondary Metabolites

Comparison of single and multitarget strategies. Proteins (represented by circles) and biomembranes (at top) are at the center of the illustration, representing molecular targets.

Wink sees a strong potential for progress in several areas, if future research is guided by an evolutionary perspective, including antimicrobial, cancer, inflammation, and gene expression.

Antimicrobial

Plant-based antimicrobial substances are less specific than modern antibiotics, which have been in use for less than sixty years. Antibiotics are fundamentally different from secondary metabolites in that they are substances that have evolved in bacteria to defend against other bacteria. Since many human pathogens have developed resistance against the specific classical antibiotics (MRSA), the search for useful plant antimicrobials with different modes of action should not be neglected.

Cancer

Plants apparently produce secondary metabolites with cytotoxic properties for animal and human cells. Whereas such compounds are usually considered toxic and are therefore avoided in phytotherapy, such secondary metabolites might be worth exploring for their ability to stop the growth of rapidly dividing cancer cells or keratocytes (skin cells), in case of psoriasis. The cytotoxic properties of secondary metabolites include permealizing biomembranes (for instance, by special classes of saponins), alkylating (adding an alkyl group such as an ethyl or methyl group) or intercalating (inserting into) DNA, or interfering with important key proteins in a cell (e.g. microtubules, DNA topoisomerase I). Cell death is usually caused by apoptosis rather than by necrosis (physiological rather than pathological causes).

Inflammation: Reactive Oxygen Species

Reactive oxygen species (ROS) are generated in the organism, but generally induced by external factors. ROS are involved in arteriosclerosis, heart disease, and aging. Secondary metabolites with conjugated double bonds (alternating single and double bonds, which allow electrons to be delocalized), such as Helichrysum, act as active radical scavengers (substances with the ability to trap or make less aggressive the unpaired electrons of free radical compounds) and can therefore be used in a broad range of indications.

Signal Transduction

A number of secondary metabolites modulate signal transduction in the neuronal network. They interact with specific receptors, ion channels, acetylcholine esterase (see essential oils for vomiting and nausea, chapter 12), protein kinase, and transporters of the presynaptic cell (which stimulate the post synaptic cell). Examples are Valerian, coffee, tea, and St. John's Wort.

Inflammation Cascade: Cyclooxygenase, Cytokines, NF-kappa Beta

A wide range of secondary metabolites is known to remedy inflammation associated with wounds, infections, or other disorders. Proteins of the inflammation cascade such as cyclooxygenase (COX) and cytokines (small proteins released from cells, which affect the behavior of other cells) are modulated by nonselective activity of secondary metabolites, causing inflammative processes to be reduced.

Gene Expression

Since proteins control the mechanisms of gene expression, the activity of secondary metabolites vis-à-vis protein targets also affects gene expression in a pleiotropic manner (with multiple effects). Diseases of the heart, circulatory and gastrointestinal systems, liver, kidney, and reproductive organs, as well as inflammation, involve the participation of several genes and proteins. While there is yet little research to provide details for this interaction, the interesting study of loggers in Scandinavia mentioned above demonstrates that their increased exposure to the terpene components of needle trees increased the expression of genes that favored increased metabolic turnover.

The Wide Reaches of Plant Medicine

By using mixtures of secondary metabolites that act on proteins and gene expression in a pleiotropic fashion, the likelihood is high that disease-relevant targets will be hit. Mixtures from plants will hit even unknown protein targets, which would not be affected by traditional monotarget therapies. Hence it is much easier to rationalize a common theme in plant medicine: the broad range of indications. This is how it is possible for us to use essential oils against inflammation and at the same time as antioxidants, antibacterials, antifungals, and antivirals.

Lavender shall serve once more as an example. Current science tells us that each component in Lavender has its own range of pleiotropic effects. Linalool, a main component of Lavender, simultaneously inhibits HMG CoA reductase (antitumor, antifungal), reduces spasms, is anticonvulsant, and modifies autonomic nervous system activity, to name only a few. These effects of linalool are then layered with at least an equal number of physiological effects of linalyl acetate, another main

From Biology to Aromatherapy

North African Essentials

Morocco is home to many aromatic and medicinal plants. Many of them, such as Rose, are cultivated and processed into absolutes by the local franchise of the perfume giants of the world. In addition there are distillers who produce such archetypical Moroccan essential oils as Atlas Cedar or the Moroccan version of Mugwort, *Artemisia herba alba*. Maybe the most coveted essential oil from Morocco for modern aromatherapy is the essential oil of *Tanacetum annuum*, Moroccan Chamomile.

Tanacetum annuum

Moroccan Chamomile, harvested in the fall, is so precious for aromatherapy because of its spectrum of sesquiterpene lactones (a large group of physiologically active sesquiterpene derivatives; lactone refers to a structural element where an ester is formed within a single molecule, resulting in a ring structure). This class of compounds inhibits a transcription factor, NF-kappa beta, which plays an important role in the cascade of events mediating inflammation. *Tanacetum annuum* apparently works at an early stage of the inflammation cascade, preventing the synthesis of the proteins that would transmit inflammation. Experience in the aromatherapy community suggests that this oil is nontoxic and its liberal addition to preparations for topical or inhalation use is free of risks.

Atlas Cedar

Atlas Cedar has all the qualities of an essential oil distilled from the core wood of a tree. It is a powerful lymphatic and arterial tonic when used topically. It is also credited with the ability to dissolve lipids and has hence become an indispensible part of cellulite preparations.

component of Lavender. In addition to the web of physiological activity present in linalool and linalyl acetate alone, there are the effects of the various monoterpene hydrocarbons. Myrcene (a common monoterpene with two double bonds), for example, acts as free radical scavenger and induces liver detoxification enzymes. This list could be continued almost indefinitely, given that over 1,200 components have been identified in Lavender essential oil. It is intuitively understandable that these layers upon layers of physiological activity of all the components in Lavender generate an overall quality, which is distinctly that of Lavender.

The vast number of processes occurring when an essential oil inter-

Understanding the
Language of Plants

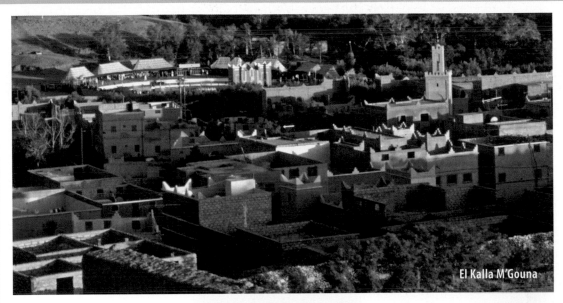

El Kalla M'Gouna

In the first week of May, La Fête de la Rose electrifies the small city of El Kalla M'Gouna in southern Morocco. Arabs, Berbers, and even some tourists from afar celebrate the harvest of the Rose (*Rosa centifolia*). A trek to this festival in El Kalla d' M'gouna has to be one of the most romantic prizes in the world of plant perfumes. For the Western traveler it is a vivid illustration of how the plant-human interface transcends even stark cultural divides.

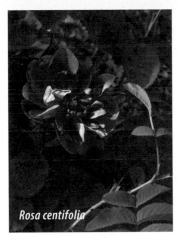

Rosa centifolia

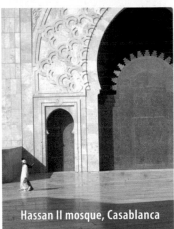

Hassan II mosque, Casablanca

acts with our bodies is best understood through the organicism perspective, which aligns the scientific process with real life's day-to-day experiences and Lavender's unrivaled ability to heal burns.

An Evolutionary Perspective on Essential Oil Activity

In the past, secondary metabolites displaying selective activity received most of the scientific attention, because their mode of action conveniently fit in to the dominant paradigm of pharmacology. Evolutionary biology and traditional healing systems show that there are many more secondary metabolites with a very broad nonselective spectrum of physiological activity.

The nonselective or pleiotropic effects of essential oils are the result of biological evolution. They arose on a time scale much larger than that of even multiple generations. Plant-human interactions, as they unfold before us, have existed since time immemorial. Cinnamon and Clove were as beneficial to humans in Hildegard von Bingen's time as they are today. This suggests a reexamination of our cherished Western notion of progress, according to which better conditions or medicines arise (only) as a result of human activity. If we want to realize the benefits of essential oils and secondary metabolites as fully as possible, we are best served by a somewhat more humble attitude.

Plant metabolites have been around for at least as long as the plants that make them. This puts the components of essential oils from gymnosperm trees—pines, conifers, and the like—at 300 million years, and the components of basically all other green plants—angiosperm plants—at approximately 100 million years. Mammalian organisms have had this entire time frame to become adjusted to and interact with the molecules of the plant world. The purportedly much safer pharmaceuticals generally are no older than fifty years. On an evolutionary time scale these synthetic drugs do not even register.

The presence of liver detoxification enzymes in the human body is one very important consequence of this very long period of continued evolutionary adjustment. Essential oil components were among the native triggers for the evolution of these enzymes. This illustrates how essential oils, with some notable exceptions, are not only not toxic but instead have unrivaled potential to induce the removal of foreign substances (such as pharmaceuticals or synthetic chemicals) from the human organism. It is ironic that our bodies would not even be able to break down and remove pharmaceuticals were it not for enzymes that evolved in response to essential oils and other secondary metabolites.

The intimate connection of essential oils to the evolution of enzymes in our own bodies is but one factor that demonstrates how essential oils have naturally, from time immemorial, interfaced with humans.

Wolves in Yellowstone

Interdependency in the natural world has resulted from millions of years of biological evolution. But we become aware of instances of interdependency only gradually, as they defy the linear notions common in our culture. A stunning example is provided by the changes occurring after the reintroduction of wolves into Yellowstone National Park. The overall result was an increase of diversity and a reappearance of other species that formerly had also become absent from this environment. As the wolves were mostly preying on elk, the latter avoided grazing in the flat river beds where they would be subject to attack more easily than in more rugged terrain. As a result, willows along the river beds, which the elk had been excessively grazing on, grew back. The increased availability of willow brought back beavers, who, by building dams and restructuring the riverbeds, brought back species that rely on wetland for their survival. This example illustrates that we may become aware of the interactions of different species sharing an environment only after we have destroyed parts of a particular environment.

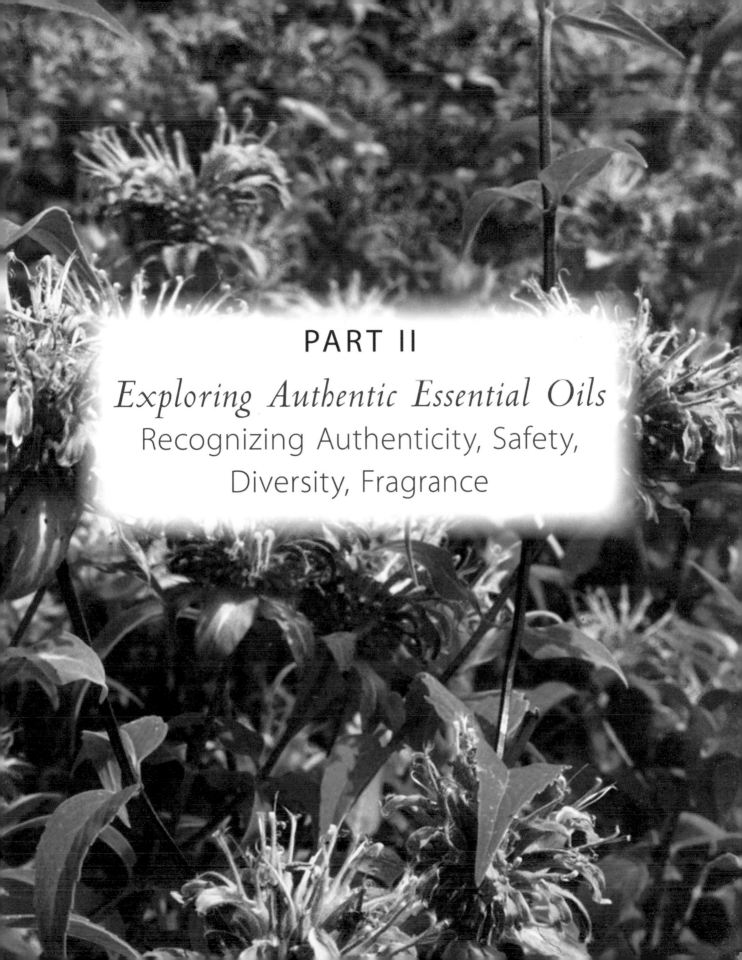

PART II

Exploring Authentic Essential Oils
Recognizing Authenticity, Safety, Diversity, Fragrance

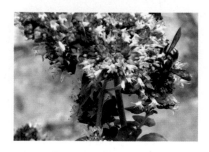

FOUR

AUTHENTIC ESSENTIAL OILS

I had always liked perfumes, but this was love.

LUCA TURIN

UNDERSTANDING AROMATHERAPY

Authenticity and Organicism

The perspectives of organicism combined with evolutionary biology provide a clear distinction of the effects of authentic and adulterated essential oils.

Authentic essential oils initiate processes designed by evolution arising at the level of the whole plant organism.

Adulterated essential oils initiate processes arising at the interface of smart engineering and the corporate objective to cut cost.

If we really intend to learn from nature, in our case from essential oils, resolving the issue of purity and authenticity is the pivot that determines whether or not we will indeed be able to learn. Considering that deception has become an integral part of economic reality in many areas of commerce, it is no surprise that it is rampant in the field of essential oils as well. An ocean of processed oils lies between the seeker and a comparatively minute quantity of truly authentic oils.

Clearly, if we use standardized essential oils, we are not learning from nature but are simply practicing more of what we already know, that technology can be used to maximize profits. Apparently limitless ingenuity is available when it comes to pawning off industrially standardized—that is, adulterated—essential oils as pure and authentic plant products. Most essential oils used for aromatherapy in the U.S. are fabrications and not genuinely and exclusively from a single plant source. As a matter of fact, the most glaring failure of the various aromatherapy organizations in the U.S. and the UK may be their inability to address the authenticity issue. Companies selling industrial and engineered essential oils penetrate these organizations and become almost indistinguishable from those who sell authentic oils.

This raises three crucial questions:

One, how can purity or absence of adulteration be ascertained?

Two, do 100 percent authentic essential oils really have effects not found in industrially standardized oils?

Three, are active ingredients responsible for the effect of the oil?

Ascertaining that an essential oil is in fact genuine and authentic is most easily accomplished by knowing its source. In an ideal situation the name of the producing company is known. Essential oil samples can then be compared to authentic samples of the producer. Nebulous statements by vendors about the origin of an essential oil typically point to industrial origin and to direct or intermediate sourcing from the Grasse or New York fragrance raw material trade. Analysis, while useful to detect gross adulterations, is generally not able to prove actual authenticity of an essential oil.

Essential Oils vs. Herbal Extracts

Research into pharmacological properties of medicinal plants often concentrates on components found in the alcohol (or water) extract. A recurrent issue in aromatherapy is the attribution of those results to the essential oil of the same plant. This is problematic, as many of the extracted molecules are different from those found in the essential oil. Frankincense essential oil is a salient example. The properties of boswellic acid, isolated from Frankincense resin by extraction, are often attributed to Frankincense essential oil, even though there is no boswellic acid in the essential oil. (See also "Frankincense" in chapter 11, page 158.)

Critics have discredited such claims as aromatherapy exuberance. From a pharmacological standpoint, there is no reason to expect the properties of the extracted, large water-soluble molecules to be identical to those found in the essential oil. Except that occasionally there is the odd observation that essential oils reflect the properties of extracts of the same plant, even though the active components of the extract are not present.

An evolutionary perspective might shed some light on this. As plants have evolved to master their challenges, their secondary metabolites, water soluble and lipophilic, all work toward the same goal. It is conceivable that lipophilic components of the plant ultimately have similar effects as the polar ones. While there is no boswellic acid in Frankincense essential oil, it is not impossible that components of the essential oil do have identical or similar properties as boswellic acid.

Standardizing or Adulterating

Standardizing and adulterating both alter the original composition of an essential oil. The difference lies in the motive. Standardization is the adjustment of an essential oil so it conforms to a given standard. This is done openly for customers who expect a specific composition.

Lavender 40/42 is a typical example. Partly or fully synthetic linalyl acetate is added to an oil so its concentration reaches between 40 and 42%! If this is done clandestinely and the customer is led to believe that it is a pure plant product, we would call this adulteration! These deceptions are often simultaneously subtle and massive. They are generally tolerated because of the misconception that natural and synthetic substances are identical if their chemical formula is identical. Adulteration is apparent in the price. It is common to find essential oils retailing for prices well below their production cost at the source. Rosemary and Lavender are prominent examples of this. Logic would dictate that this is only possible by extension with less expensive materials.

Authentic Essential Oils

Exploring the Gardens of the Unadulterated

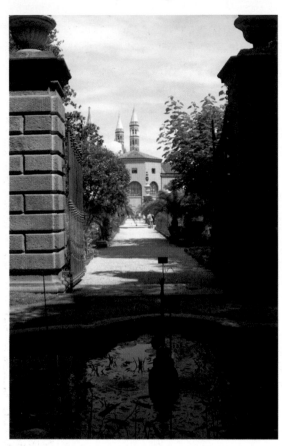

The Orto Botanico at the University of Padua

The botanical garden of the University of Padua illustrates the multidimensionality of plant-human relations. Founded in the year 1545, it is the oldest academic botanical garden in the world. In the middle of the sixteenth century there was great uncertainty about the proper identification of the medicinal plants of antiquity as they had been used by famous healers such Hippocrates (ca. 460 BCE–ca. 370 BCE) of Greece, considered the father of Western medicine, and Galen (ca. 129 CE–ca. 217 CE), a prominent Roman physician, surgeon, and philosopher. Accidents and fraud were common, with sometimes dire consequences for public health. A decree of the Republic of Venice (the Serenissima) mandated the cultivation of medicinal plants, or, as they were called, the "unadulterated ones." *Unadulterated* was the term used for medicines that came directly from nature. Plants were by

The concept of organicism has important repercussions for our understanding of the activity of authentic essential oils as opposed to the common commercial products engineered by the big brokerage firms. As pharmacology is limited to molecular phenomena, it has no measure for authenticity. From the perspective of organicism, it is reasonable to assume that the physiological effects triggered by authentic essential oils are an expression of the whole plant organism striving for survival and successful reproduction, and not just a combination of components.

Authentic essential oils feature a set of secondary metabolites that have proven most effective through the trials of biological evolution.

far the largest group of unadulterated medicines; others may have been minerals and animal products. For this very reason the first botanical gardens were called "Gardens of the Unadulterated" (*Hortus Simplicium*).

The original layout of the garden had the medicinal plants arranged in a way that reflected the complex mathematical and astrological systems of medieval medicine. To this day the garden remains an invaluable resource for the study of these forms of astrological geography and plant medicine.

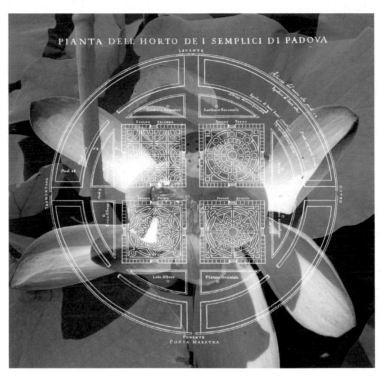

Apparently the patricians of Venice relied heavily on the various species of Lotus. The Orto Botanico features a wide variety of water lilies, such as this one on which the layout of the garden is superimposed.

Even in authentic essential oils the original composition of secondary metabolites is already modified by chemical reactions that happen during distillation. But in the commercial oils, even though they are often constructed from isolated natural materials rather than synthetics, the original intent, the original evolutionary design that makes a Rosemary oil the representation of that plant, is lost.

There is also the philosophical issue of how an essential oil can be Rosemary oil when its components were previously isolated from Eucalyptus and Orange. In addition, there are manifest material differences. While the components isolated from Eucalyptus and used to reconstruct Rosemary may be identical in name, often secondary features

Authentic Essential Oils

Adulteration in Detail

"The Adulteration of Essential Oils and the Consequences to Aromatherapy and Natural Perfumery" is a comprehensive and most informed review of industrial essential oil adulteration by Tony Burfield. In it, Burfield lists the principal ways in which oils can be adulterated and, oil by oil, gives the specific adulterants employed. It is a must-read for anyone who wants to understand the true scope of the phenomenon.[1]

such as stereochemistry or isomer ratios are different. As a result, using reconstructed Rosemary essential oil, as most users in Western aromatherapy do, will deliver some effects inherent in the components mixed together in the oil. But the life-supporting qualities emerging at the level of the whole Rosemary organism are missing.

The perspective of organicism also illustrates how essential oils from wild plants can be fundamentally different from those distilled from cultivated plants. This is not to say that essential oils from wild plants are always better; they simply reflect a different status and sensitivity of the plant organism. The oil from a wild plant reflects the plant's efforts to survive on its own, whereas the oil distilled from cultivated plants reflects, at least to a degree, the intention and intervention of the growers to obtain a favorable fragrance and a good yield. A phenomenon often observed in viticulture is also observed in growing essential oil plants: the stresses of the environment are reflected in the spectrum of fragrant molecules the plant produces. Essential oils from wild plants do not necessarily have a stronger fragrance, but they show increased complexity and, subjectively, more elegance.

The Mechanics of Essential Oil Standardization

The purpose of industrial standardization is to bring the essential oils to a price point deemed acceptable. This is done by adding low molecular monoterpene components that are nonsuspicious because they are already present in the oil and therefore not readily detectable as adulterants. These monoterpenoid add-ons are generally isolated from less expensive oils and are available inexpensively on the market. For example, the molecule linalool is present in an authentic Lavender oil. Adding a little bit more linalool from another source, synthetic or natural, will not automatically raise a red flag; superficially, nothing grossly foreign has been added.

If this process is repeated for a number of prominent monoterpene components in an oil, the relative proportions of its main components may even remain similar to the original. Yet by increasing the concentration of the main components, the trace components, with their specific physiological activity, will have been reduced in their concentration from very low to practically zero. The presence or absence of these trace components is a common, major difference between industrial and authentic essential oils.

Are Adulterated Essential Oils Still Active?

Then the question arises regarding how authenticity—or the lack thereof—reflects on the therapeutic efficacy of essential oils. As is often the case in real life, the answers are not black and white. Whether purists like it or not, there are, in fact, therapeutic applications of essential oils, such as those for herpes, that can be quite successful even with oils that are not 100 percent authentic. But for other treatments, especially for metabolic and degenerative diseases, where many different components of the essential oil interact simultaneously with multiple systems in the body, success appears to hinge entirely on the authenticity of the chosen oils.

Three Layers of Activity

An explanation for the observation that sometimes almost any oil will do and at other times only a truly authentic oil will show activity lies in the fact that essential oils display at least three general types of physiological activity.

The most common type of activity is nonselective.[2] Nonselective activity is generally encountered in the low molecular, lipophilic monoterpenes present in almost all essential oils. These components are stimulant, antibacterial, and antiviral, and they also modify the cell membrane. Antiviral activity appears to be a nonselective quality of essential oils. For example, herpes can be treated with almost every essential oil from Anise to Xanthoxyllum. This is a consequence of the evolutionary modeling that favored the components that protected the plant from as many challenges as possible.

A second type of essential oil activity is selective in nature. Selective or specific effects have been attributed mostly to larger, somewhat more complex constituents, such as sesquiterpenes, diterpenes, and sesquiterpene lactones, which, as we have seen, often interact with specific cellular processes.

Third, there is the combined effect of all the nonselective and the selective components of a specific plant species acting in unison to

Henri Viaud

Henry Viaud was the grand seigneur of distilling essential oils for the purpose of aromatherapy. He was the first to articulate that an essential oil for aromatherapy needed to fulfill a different set of criteria than those for the fragrance industry. He stated that essential oils had to be "genuine and authentic" in order to be acceptable for aromatherapy.

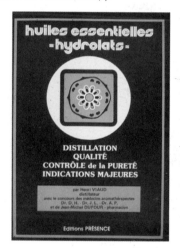

generate its characteristic effect. The totality of all the components interacts with many or all of our organ systems exactly as modeled by the evolution of that particular plant. This fine-tuned multidimensional effect of the natural composition produced by evolution cannot be duplicated by clever mixing of components in a lab. The chromatograms (analyses) that are often presented to demonstrate the identical composition of the original natural oil and its artificial copy are only crude approximations. They can do nothing to account for the many physical, chemical, and biological differences between the two.

In the language of biology, the qualities typically associated with Rosemary or Lavender oil emerge at the organizational level of the whole plant organism. No single component or mixture of components has been found that will duplicate the power of Lavender oil to heal burns. Another example is provided by Greenland Moss: the whole oil lowers pathologically elevated liver enzyme counts, but none of its isolated components will do the same. Yet another example for the unexpected effectiveness of authentic essential oils is the balancing of premenstrual progesterone deficiency with *Vitex agnus castus*. Practically every woman in the aromatherapy community who has used this essential oil will attest to its powerful effects. Apparently there is a combination of selective activity of some sesqui- and diterpenes as well as an emerging quality of the whole oil in which selective effects team up with the nonselective effects of the ubiquitous monoterpenes to produce the distinct effects of *Vitex agnus castus* essential oil.

Summing up, it can be understood that essential oils, even if they are standardized or adulterated, will display the nonselective effects of commonly present monoterpene components, such as an antiviral effect. However, selective effects due to specific sesquiterpenes generally disappear with standardization.

Most importantly, the complete effect—the properties emerging at the level of the whole organism expressing the characteristic qualities of a specific species—are woefully absent from doctored oils. As the adulterants do not originate from the living plant but from a man-made laboratory, they express the characteristics of the latter.

Degrees of Authenticity: Eucalyptus radiata *and* Eucalyptus globulus

The idea that the essential oil of the whole plant organism transcends the limited narrative of its chemical composition can be experienced with our senses.

Eucalyptus oils have been homogenized as a result of the recognition of 1.8 cineole (a ubiquitous terpenoid essential oil constituent) as an expectorant agent. Commercial Eucalyptus oils smell and feel like . . . Eucalyptus oil. The redistillation (one phase distillation of an essential oil intended to separate desired from undesired components) of Eucalyptus oils to produce the commercial cineole-enriched form reduces them to the molecular plane. The fragrance of an authentic sample of *Eucalyptus radiata,* however, reflects the whole organism. It is dramatically different and more complex. Comparing commercial Eucalyptus with authentic *Eucalyptus radiata* juxtaposes the one-dimensional sting of an isolated component (1.8 cineole) with the undomesticated fragrance of a specific plant species.

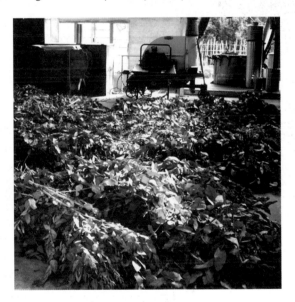

The leaves of one-year-old *Eucalyptus globulus* are round and have not yet assumed their adult longish shape. This difference in morphology makes it easy to distill essential oils from distinctly different points in the life cycle of the tree. We can recognize distinct differences between the fragrance of an authentic essential oil of an adult plant and that of a one-year-old Eucalyptus.

Both *Eucalyptus radiata* and *Eucalyptus globulus* are nontoxic and are most advantageously used topically and for inhalation.

Essential Oil Composition: Inevitably Variable

Biology is the science of life. It is more interested in describing the phenomena of living organisms than bending those phenomena to the need of a specific industry. Biology recognizes that essential oils distilled from different populations of identical species reflect the response of the plant metabolism to prevailing environmental conditions. The genetic

The Aromatic Language of Corsica

Corsica is the cradle of medical aromatherapy. On this island the unique combination of plants, climate, and culture led to the development of the pioneering distillation operations that devoted themselves exclusively to the aromatherapy market.

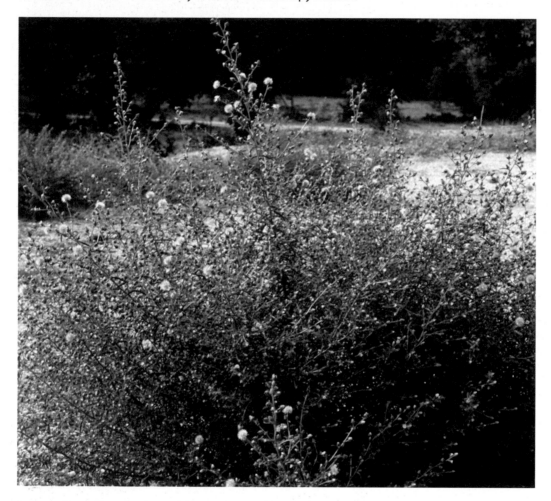

Inula graveolens was given early recognition in *L'aromatherapie exactement* as one of the strongest mucolytic essential oils. It counteracts candida in the bronchial system and tonifies the heart. It has become an aromatherapy highlight through a combination of factors. It is indeed a highly effective mucolytic agent. When passed around on a smell strip during a seminar, slight coughing and throat clearing will ensue. It has been used in French aromatherapy to soften hardened mucus and to initiate lung cleansing.

The second factor is clearly coincidental. When the essential oil of *Inula graveolens* started its triumphant expansion into the world, the still in which it was extracted was copper. Apparently some trace components in this oil form complexes with copper and, voilà, the essential oil turns out emerald green. Distilled in stainless steel it is yellowish clear! It is best used sparingly—a drop on your sleeping pillow is quite effective.

The essential oil and fragrance of *Lentiscus pistachius* or Mastick is alluring in more than one way. It is one of the fragrances mentioned in the Gilgamesh epic from Mesopotamia, one of the earliest known works of literature on planet Earth. Its therapeutics are determined by its astringent character; it is a formidable decongestant for lymph, veins, and prostate. The nonirritant and nontoxic quality of this oil encourage the interested individual to explore liberally.

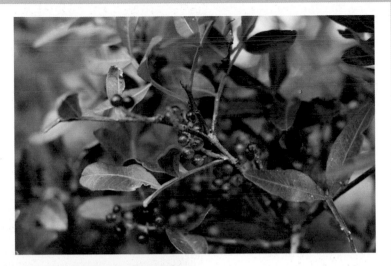

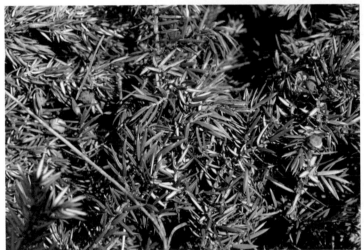

The oil of *Juniperus communis* var. *montana,* or Mountain Juniper, is naturally high in limonene and almost free of sabinene, the terpene hydrocarbon most prone to irritate the kidneys. Obtaining authentic Juniper essential oils is not always easy. The Corsican variety of Mountain Juniper has an exquisite, crisp aroma, its sublime fragrance testifying to the difference between the common soup and authentic oil. The oil is anti-inflammative and analgesic. It has an interesting resonance with the nervous system, easing neuralgic pain as well as balancing the autonomic nervous system.

The essential oil of *Myrtus communis* from Corsica is referred to as Green Myrtle in aromatherapy. The oil from North Africa is brownish in color and has a rather different composition. Green Myrtle is of high therapeutic value. It is most useful for all respiratory conditions, especially those involving not just the bronchial tracts but also the lungs themselves. It is extremely gentle and can be used liberally. Green Myrtle is also helpful for hypothyroidism.

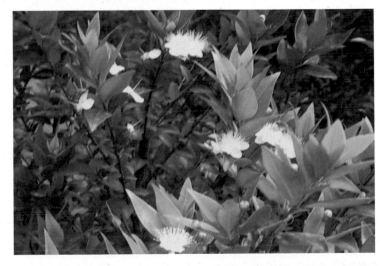

Thymus vulgaris: *Chemical Chameleon*

When the phenomenon of chemotypes first gained traction in aromatherapy, the impression arose that they were distinct entities or some form of subspecies. This was probably due to the authoritative numbering by French authors, such as calling Thyme linalool CT one, Thyme geraniol CT two, and so on.

Closer examination shows that this impression also arose because growers would clone Thyme plants whose attractive fragrance promised a desirable composition, for instance a high concentration of linalool. The grower would make clippings, multiply the plant, and thereby be able to distill an oil with a composition matching that of the original.

The wild progenitors of these cloned plants thrive on the slopes of Provence, where the composition of their essential oil may vary dramatically from plant to plant. In addition, distinct populations have evolved in locked-in valleys with chemical compositions all their own.

For quite some time now, there have been producers distilling Thyme gathered in the wild, in other words "population Thyme." These oils provide the closest representation of the set of secondary metabolites with which the Thyme plants respond to the differences in altitude and the corresponding variation of energy in the spectrum of visible light (shorter wavelength blue light is more energetic than longer wavelength red light). As with Lavender, essential oils of wild Thyme are lighter and softer than the oils from the cloned plants.

Thymus vulgaris of the paracymene type is gathered in the wild at elevations slightly above sea level. It is a most interesting and useful variety. Paracymene is the compound immediately preceding thymol in its biosynthesis. In plants growing at even lower altitudes, biosynthesis runs through to the last step: paracymene adds on a hydroxyl group (the -OH structural element) and turns into the irritant thymol or carvacrol. Thyme paracymene is a stimulant but not too irritant. According to French aromatherapy, it is used topically for arthritis. It is also a most effective antibacterial agent. This oil has power, but it does not burn.

program of the plant species codes for the biochemical machinery and the range of components it could potentially synthesize. The specific conditions a population faces determine which subset of the whole chemical arsenal of metabolites available to them is in fact activated.

For example, camphor apparently supports *Rosmarinus officina-*

Populations that yield Thyme oils rich in the terpene alcohol thuyanol grow in the area surrounding Nice and on the slopes of the Pyrenees. *Thymus vulgaris* of the thuyanol type also is nontoxic and nonirritating, with a most outstanding antiviral and antibacterial efficacy. Ingesting up to 5 drops of this oil 3 or 4 times per day to avoid oncoming infections has been done without any undesirable side effects. It is also well tolerated by most individuals on the mucous membranes of the sexual organs to counteract or prevent viral or bacterial infection. Thyme thuyanol combines the mild qualities of the high altitude linalool and geraniol types with the antiviral and antibacterial vigor of the more aggressive oils of the lower elevations.

The linalool and geraniol types of *Thymus vulgaris* are the most ethereal Thyme oils. They convey much of the antimicrobial strength of the oils of the lower elevations, but they are extremely mild and also fragrant. They are the antiseptic agents of choice for skincare.

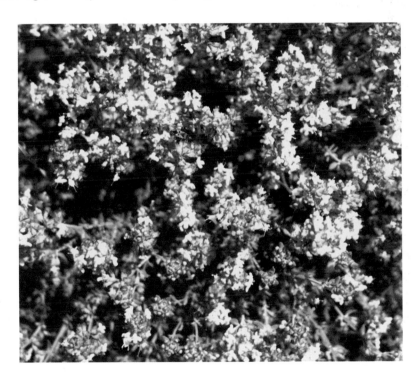

Thyme thuyanol cultivated 20 miles inland of Nice, at an altitude of about 2,300 feet

lis in its quest to survive and reproduce at higher altitudes. Rosemary from the high plateaus of Provence has up to 20 percent camphor, while Rosemary growing at sea level produces no camphor. Authentic samples of essential oil of Rosemary harvested in coastal areas of California, Corsica, Croatia, or Haute Provence differ significantly in their

Adulteration and
Allergies

The perspective of evolutionary biology explains why authentic oils almost never cause allergies and why adulterated oils do.

When the human body encounters an authentic essential oil it encounters a mix of substances it has known for very long—evolutionary—periods of time. When our bodies encounter adulterated oils, the substances in the mix are slightly or even drastically different from what our bodies have adapted to throughout evolution. Our bodies are unfamiliar with these substances and their mixtures and begin to release histamine to flush out the foreign substances.

respective content of cineole, camphor, bornyl acetate, and verbenone. Samples with low camphor and high verbenone contents are referred to as "Rosemary verbenone" (California, Corsica). This oil has been recognized for its specific mucolytic qualities and its usefulness for skin care formulas. The Haute Provence variety with high cineole and high camphor content is used in aromatherapy for asthenia as well as for its expectorant and anti-infectious effects.[3] Rosemary essential oil from the islands off the Adriatic coast of Croatia has a composition squarely in the middle, with a camphor content of approximately 10 percent. It appears that there really are not distinct chemotypes, such as a "verbenone type" or "Spanish type," but simply Rosemary essential oils with higher or lower camphor content.

As plants change with the seasons, so does their production of secondary metabolite defenses. The composition of a plant's essential oil changes continuously during its life cycle. The essential oil produced to protect young leafy shoots will be different from the one stored in the seed. It also varies between different organs of the plant and between individuals of a population. This constant change in composition is reflected in truly authentic essential oils. Different from standardized essential oils required for industrial production processes, authentic essential oils reflect the seasonal and climatic variation of nature, changing from year to year or from harvest to harvest. This constant variation has strong ecological advantages. Experience has shown that the development of resistance is only an attribute of single component drugs with specific single modes of action!

However, the fact that essential oil composition is subject to perpetual variation presents a conceptual problem for pharmacology. If two essential oils, for instance two distillates from two *Thymus vulgaris* populations, have different chemical composition, they are liable, at least within the context of conventional pharmacology, to have different pharmacological effects. But for medicinal purposes, only essential oils with a specific and known composition—the ones for which all the tests were conducted—are admissible.

This led to the practice of standardizing extracts. But standardizing comes with a price: it diminishes authenticity and sometimes serves as a pretext for outright adulteration. This practice went so far that certain extracts were standardized for a specific component, such as hypericin in St. John's Wort, even though everyone admitted that hypericin was not responsible for the plant's effects. This is just one example of the contortions that have to be made when complexity is described with reductionism.

An interesting note is that while hypericin is, together with hyperforin, one of the principal constituents of the plant of *Hypericum perforatum,* St. John's Wort, due to its high molecular weight, it is not present in the essential oil.

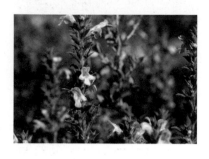

FIVE

AROMATHERAPY SAFETY IN THE INFORMATION AGE

While I was here last September, I got sick as a consequence of my work. I was picking tomatoes near Oxnard. My fingernails became infected as a result of the poison that was on the tomato plants. Some of my fingernails fell off.

ANONYMOUS BRACERO QUOTED BY LINDA NASH
IN *INESCAPABLE ECOLOGIES*

If one is new to aromatherapy, the safety of essential oil use is a crucial factor. But much of what has been written about it is simply wrong, which makes it difficult for the novice to get a clear picture. Here we shall try to dispel the various myths that intentionally or unintentionally inflate the dangers of essential oils and identify the interests that put the myths in place.

Most notably the fragrance industry projected its own concerns—which are starkly different from those of aromatherapy—into this debate. In the 1970s and 1980s an almost irrational alarmism was fanned by the surrogates of this industry. The motives behind this campaign were generally those of an industry engaged in turf battles. The factual arguments were clearly pseudoscientific, operating from the obsolete paradigm that essential oils were random mixtures of potentially unknown and treacherous chemicals.

Many industry and academic experts at the time maintained that safety could only be established by subjecting essential oils and their components to the same tests as commercial skin care or perfume products. These statements received disproportionate attention, not so much for their scientific value, but for the controversial tone in which they were presented. When essential oils were actually tested with the methods of the skin care industry, the results were inconclusive, thereby reflecting the basic misunderstanding of the nature of essential oils.

Topics not factually connected to essential oil safety were thrown in the stew to make it even more cloudy. For example, fragrance industry guidelines that exaggerate the hazards of natural materials and trivialize those of synthetics were often used to overstate the hazards of essential oils.

In a related development, the art of the disclaimer reached new levels of perfection. A particularly pointless example, repeated in book after book, was the admonition that essential oils should only be ingested under the supervision of a licensed physician—when all the authors were keenly aware that there were only a handful of conventional physicians who knew anything about essential oils.

The pointless mantra about supervision by a licensed practitioner illustrates the eager subordination of authors to the conventional system. This contorted mindset first contends that the conventional medical process is the gold standard where everything is always safe and perfect. Starting with this patently wrong assumption makes it possible to exaggerate the slightest concern with respect to essential oils. At one time the literature was full of warnings that essential oils might precipitate epileptic seizures. If this had been true, the watchdogs of industrial medicine, always present to discredit plant medicine, justified or not, would have certainly amplified the concern.

Then came the dire warnings about the use of Cinnamon and Clove oil. "Never to be used" was a favorite phrase attached to these two essential oils, which was, however, resoundingly ignored by those who really used essential oils. The antibacterial effects of Cinnamon Bark oil make it one of the best options when a person encounters violent bacterial infections of the intestinal tract, especially while traveling in unfamiliar territory! The choice is between being pointlessly scared by the defensive writing of an author who probably had never been in a comparable situation or effectively ending the debilitating condition with a few drops of Cinnamon oil.

A thorough analysis of the many and varied contributions to the discourse about essential oil safety could fill a volume of mainly sarcastic diatribes. To acquire the necessary degree of comfort and ease

In the 1970s and 1980s a substantial number of monographs on fragrance raw materials were published in the journal *Food and Cosmetics Toxicology*.[1]

These toxicology tests were generated by and for the fragrance industry. By default they reproduced the biases of that industry. The operative paradigm held that because of the random nature of fragrant plant substances no assumptions could be made about their general safety and that all essential oil components had to be properly vetted before allowing public use. During the early years of modern aromatherapy these studies became something of a secret weapon for those who argued that much more science was needed.

Aromatherapy Safety in the Information Age

when using essential oils, we shall adopt a more relaxed attitude, trying to look through the many bogus warnings of nonexistent dangers, while cultivating an awareness of a very short list of real hazards.

Ultimately, an assessment of the literature that deals with the potential toxicity of essential oils reveals that those oils typically used in aromatherapy have not even been investigated. Most warnings are derived from industry-funded dermatological tests with limited relevance for aromatherapy.

The reader will find that basic information and a dose of common sense are a perfect foundation to safely explore the many uses of essential oils. This is not to say that there will never be an unpleasant experience. An oil might be irritating or more stimulating than expected. But it is also possible to view these experiences as manifestations of a renewed physiological bond with nature.

Compared to the hundreds of thousands of deaths caused by the wrongful application of conventional medicines and the hundreds of thousands more deaths caused by known side effects of conventional drugs, the journeys to explore essential oils are innocent and utterly harmless.

Why Natural Is Safer After All

If being in harmony with nature provides a sound basis for well-being, it might immediately follow that natural substances—natural medicines—are inherently safer than synthetic drugs. This notion has been fought tooth and nail by the representatives of chemical, pharmaceutical, fragrance, flavor, and food industries.

The official view contends that there is no difference between natural and so-called nature identical substances (synthesized in the laboratory and considered identical to those that occur in nature, because superficially they have the same structural formula as their natural counterparts) and that a preference for natural materials arises from irrational herd behavior of consumers conned into green trends. For instance, the alcohol linalool from a plant is considered to be identical and equivalent to the same alcohol linalool made in the laboratory, since they share the same molecular formula. This is, however, not true. There are significant physical, biological, and ultimately chemical differences between the two. (For a detailed explanation, please refer to my book *Aromatherapy Lifestyle.*[4])

Further, the industry line maintains that natural substances come with many dubious impurities and that pure, industrial single-substance products are much safer. The latter contention is also misleading, as industrial molecules are also never 100 percent pure; their impurities are simply different from those in nature and potentially much more toxic.

While it would be naive to believe that every natural molecule is safe and every synthetic is somehow evil, the fact is that the above reasoning is a gross—and knowing—distortion of the truth. The safety of natural medicines is exponentially higher than that of synthetic drugs, according to whichever statistic is examined. Arguments that complete essential oils can be less toxic than isolated components have been discussed as early as in R. Tisserand's 1988 *Essential Oil Safety Data Manual.*[5]

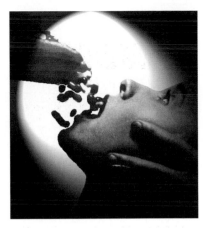

The safety statistics of conventional medicine are murderous.

Turning the Argument from Its Head onto Its Feet

To get out from underneath these layers of trumped-up concerns, the whole safety and toxicity discussion needs to be turned upside down. Instead of perpetuating mantras about imaginary dangers, the inherently benign nature of essential oils needs to be recognized.

As we have seen, many misconceptions arose from the "chemistry only" perspective, which implied that essential oils are mixtures of random chemicals derived by distillation of plant material. The operative word here is *random,* because it implies that nothing can be said a priori about the benign or toxic character of these substances and that safety and toxicity have to be determined case by case, molecule by molecule, through the tireless efforts of the chemists in the fragrance, flavor, and pharmaceutical industries. But, as we have seen, the biological perspective reveals that in reality the components of essential oils are not random; they instead reflect the evolution and environment of the living plant organisms from which they are distilled. Looking at natural multicomponent mixtures as if they were random chemicals is simply obsolete.

Experience Contradicts Hyped Concerns

Consequently many aromatherapy rules based on the assumption of random toxicity are not justified by any perceivable reality. For example, many texts will decree never to use essential oils undiluted, when in fact quite a number of essential oils can safely be used undiluted on the skin.

The same is true for ingesting essential oils. Outlawed in many texts, ingesting a drop of essential oil is generally nothing more than an experience characterized by strong turpentine flavor sensations, but not by imminent danger. Certain essential oils that have been relegated by some authors into the "should not be used at all" category are some of the therapeutically most useful.

Even the "safety of essential oils during pregnancy" discussion seems to abate due to the stubborn absence of reports of any adverse effects. And the much-feared potential of Rosemary oil to induce seizures has so far failed to throw all of Britain into a collective state of epilepsy.

Undesirable Effects of Essential Oils

Developing a sense for the real side effects of essential oils is something that every lay individual with a modicum of common sense will easily accomplish. Many of the warnings found in the literature are readily recognized as defensive attitude mandated by publishers instructing their authors. At the same time, some essential oils can be toxic when used wrongly. It is imperative to be able to recognize these essential oils and either avoid them or take the necessary precautions when working with them.

Watching for Essential Oils with Ketones

Some essential oils contain components called ketones (the ketone group is a structural element in which oxygen is bound to a carbon by a double bond), which can be toxic, and some essential oils contain nontoxic ketones, such as the verbenone in Rosemary verbenone. Here we shall concentrate on those essential oils whose specific ketone components can be a hazard.

Identifying these essential oils is not that complicated, as there are only a few in general circulation: Sage, Mugwort, Thuja, *Hyssop officinalis,* and *Lavandula stoechas.* Ingesting 3 drops of any of these oils constitutes an excessive dose with potentially serious toxicity. These oils should either be avoided or only used if you are familiar with the proper ways to use them despite their toxicity. Detailed literature on this topic is readily available (see, for example, my book *Advanced Aromatherapy*[6]).

Sage (*Salvia officinalis*) is grown in many parts of the world. Its outstanding chemical characteristic is its high content of the monoterpene ketone thujone. As an isolated substance, thujone is undoubtedly toxic. It imparts its liver and nerve toxicity to oils such as Thuja (*Thuja occidentalis*) and Mugwort (*Artemisia herbe alba*). Oddly enough, toxicity tests have shown that Sage essential oil is less toxic than what would be expected, based on its normal thujone content of over 40 percent. In addition, distilling Sage (*Salvia officinalis*) early in its life cycle, when the leaves are still very small, yields an oil with very low thujone content.

Watching for Essential Oils That Are Skin Irritants

There are some essential oils that are outright irritants and others that can cause skin irritation under certain circumstances. Awareness of these possibilities is easy to gain and simple to act upon.

Peroxidization

Essential oils may become peroxidized for a number of reasons and consequently contain irritant peroxide components. This phenomenon is a bit puzzling, as peroxides may be irritant even though they are only present in the most minute trace concentrations, significantly below 1 percent of the whole oil. The way to minimize this problem is to know that it is, according to current knowledge, most prevalent with citrus, needle, and Tea Tree oils. Even if an essential oil is normally known as

Ketones

Sage

Enterprising distillers have found a way around the high ketone content in Sage essential oil. Distilling Sage (*Salvia officinalis*) early in its life cycle, when the leaves are still very small, yields an oil with very low thujone content.

To become familiar with the way in which these differences are reflected in the fragrance, compare Dalmatian Sage, which has a characteristic thujone note, with the fragrance of the small leaf Sage oil (*Sauge petite feuilles*).

Hyssop officinalis and *Hyssop decumbens*

Hyssop officinalis is valued for its beneficial effects on the respiratory system and the relief it can provide asthma sufferers. However, it contains a significant proportion of the ketone pinocamphone, which makes it difficult or impossible to exploit the beneficial effects of this oil.

In the past, distillers in Provence wildcrafted an essential oil from *Hyssop officinalis* var. *decumbens*. More recently *Hyssopus off.* var. *montana intermedia* has been cultivated in its place. This variety has a very low or no ketone content, yet it still has all the benefits for the respiratory tract. It can safely be used for many different conditions and is, because of its mild and nontoxic nature, even well suited for children. While the essential oil is extremely mild it is also strongly antiviral.

As a nontoxic, powerful antiviral *Hyssop decumbens* (*Hyssopus off.* var. *montana intermedia*) can be used for adults and infants. It can be dabbed undiluted on herpes lesions or fever blisters inside the mouth. It is an excellent component in synergies for sinusitis and bronchitis. As a respectable sympathotonic, the oil eases nervous depression, anxiety, and asthma-related symptoms. To explore, use it in the shower or integrate it into a lotion!

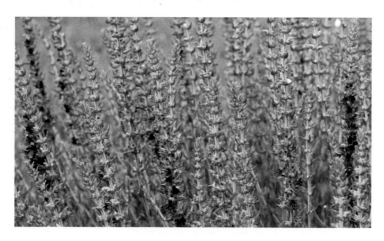

Hyssop decumbens (properly referred to as *Hyssopus off.* var. *montana intermedia*) cultivated near Banon. This Hyssop is safe to use. Unlike the *officinalis* variety, it is free of hazardous ketones.

Approaching the Stronger Oils from the Tropics

Cinnamon and Clove

The potential of the essential oils of these two plants to induce sensitization and consequently allergic reactions has been at the center of controversy. The fact is that for individuals with a corresponding disposition these essential oils do present significant hazards. Those who follow the edicts of British-style aromatherapy often choose never to touch these essential oils. Another course of action is to explore your own susceptibility to these essential oils. One way to do this is to put the most minute fraction of a drop on the skin inside the elbow.

It appears that the potential of Clove bud, stem, and leaf as well as Cinnamon bark and leaf oil to create these undesirable effects arises when they come in contact with the skin. However, ingesting a drop of Cinnamon Bark essential oil absorbed on a sugar cube or a similar adsorbent is typically tolerated well by almost everyone. Taking a drop of Cinnamon Bark essential oil in this fashion can be a life safer if you are suffering from tropical infections.

Clove essential oil is so powerful that it is treated with utmost respect by everyone who chooses to work with it. If integrated into blends intended for ingestion, 1% of Clove is effective and should probably be an upper limit.

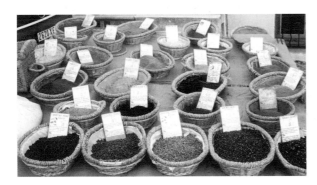

Spices at a market in Provence

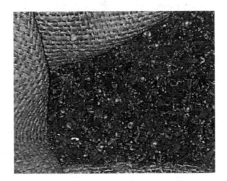

Cloves in the Sampoerna Cigarette Factory in Surabaya

Palmarosa

Palmarosa essential oil originally comes from India and Pakistan. It is nontoxic and its opulent, yet still very attractive, geraniol-dominated fragrance signals its connection to hotter climates. It has been described as effective for tropical infections. Palmarosa is best used topically but can, in conjunction with other oils, also be ingested.

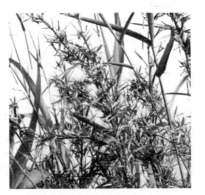

Palmarosa

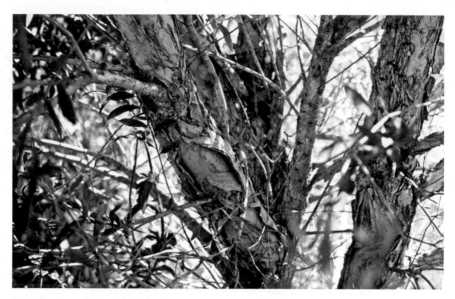

Paperbark tree (*Melaleuca quinquenervia viridiflora*)

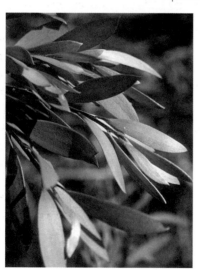

Paperbark tree leaves

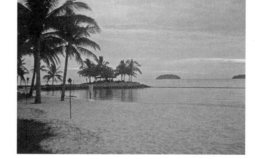

Sunset in Sabah

The Paperbark tree, or Niaouli, brings Southern Hemisphere vitality to the world.

Niaouli/Paperbark Tree

The Paperbark tree, *Melaleuca quinquenervia viridiflora,* originates from the Indonesian archipelago and northern Australia. Today the bulk of the Niaouli essential oil on the market comes from Madagascar. The oil is a typical expression of the Myrtaceae character. It is very effective in strengthening the immune response. It is best used by applying a few drops to the skin in the shower (see page 126) or in blends to prevent or address upper respiratory conditions. For its use in preventing radiation burns, see page 185.

nonirritant, if you experience it as an irritant you can simply avoid it or use it only for diffusing.

Sensitization

Sensitization is a process that leads to an overshooting immune response. With respect to essential oils this means they might be tolerated initially but can cause disproportionately strong dermatitis reactions with subsequent uses, even in response to minute concentrations. Some oils, especially Cinnamon (bark and leaf) and Clove (bud, stem, and leaf), statistically have the capacity to sensitize more than others. If used on the skin in concentrations above 2 percent, Cinnamon and Clove are considered irritant, meaning they will elicit an inflammation response from everyone, not just those who have become sensitized to them. Most interestingly, these effects are related to topical application; it appears, from experience in the aromatherapy community, that the internal application does not carry the same risks. A large body of literature exists for those who wish to study this topic more thoroughly.

Irritation

Some components of essential oils and certain whole essential oils will irritate everyone's skin if applied in a high enough concentration. Generally irritant essential oils are those with phenolic components: Thyme thymol, Oregano, and Savory. However, almost any oil can be an irritant to specific individuals based on their unique disposition. The continued use of the same oil may also, over time, lead to irritation not experienced when the oil was first tried out.

Aromatherapy in the Information Age

We face several different influences as we make decisions about whether to choose conventional treatment or natural healing. Personal factors are tantamount for these decisions, as we sometimes deal with deeper cultural and philosophical issues than is convenient to admit. These philosophical and cultural aspects tend to remain subconscious as a consequence of the way we process and value information.

Through the digital revolution, information has become the currency of almost everything. As with money, so with information: more is better. To learn about the merits of a therapeutic modality, we collect

Drugs consist of single components, they bypass sensory evaluation, and they almost make our chemical senses obsolete; therefore drug activity is proven by data sets, perceived as hard science and real information.

Natural medicines consist of complex mixtures; their effects are proven by experience, anecdotes, and traditional information.

information and ask for scientific evidence. We seek answers through TV, print, and Internet. We keep collecting and accumulating, and when it is time to analyze, assess, and evaluate, we are instead inundated with more information. According to arguments outlined in Theodore Roszak's *Cult of Information,* compiling and processing information increasingly substitutes for thinking. The information overflow makes it hard to detect intentional falsification by omission.

Looking on the Internet for science related to a specific remedy is particularly telling. There seems to be an accepted code for how different websites are supposed to look. From FDA-approved drugs to science-based supplements to pure hippie-esque herbal remedies, each category has its own stylistic language. The single component drugs developed by corporate pharmacology have official-looking sites with stern and authoritative language, invoking the feel of a government site. Information about herbal products, to the contrary, is displayed on more colorful and relaxed sites in less militaristic language.

Most of us will subconsciously accept the insinuated conclusion: single component drugs must be really effective, since their websites exude authority. Multicomponent drugs and nutraceuticals are clearly less serious, which is proven by the design of their websites. Empiricism, traditional medicines, and intuitive approaches are suppressed by the way the metaphysics of information makes us value abstract data sets of corporate science over our own experiences and sensory perceptions.

Plant Information, Media Commercials, and Data Sets

Ponder, for a moment, the different qualities of information contained in biomolecules and commercial drugs. Essential oils speak to our sense of smell, we see their color, and their texture is apparent to the touch. Pharmacology constructs its drugs to work in ways hidden from our senses, alleging that their effects are best detected by the devices of the internist! We accept that the chemical senses that have served us well throughout evolution are no longer to be trusted. We accept manipulation of our mental plane as a substitute.

Where essential oils generate a broadband symphony for our senses, feeding the vital plane of consciousness, drugs only speak to our senses indirectly through text and images generated by advertising agencies. A TV ad uses our senses of hearing and seeing to feed the mental plane. Drug propaganda—lacking any vital element—is rationalized by our dominant culture of science, with its implied human superiority over nature.

Scientism

The purported foundation of drug efficacy in rational science is belied by its own storytelling: ads for corporate drugs typically portray humans rendered pain free and happy by the blessings of science. At the same time, most lay individuals have no way of comprehending the referenced science. Instead, we believe in science. Our language reflects this too: "They (sic!!) found out that . . ." We use the nebulous "they" whenever we refer to what we believe to be scientific fact. Science has become the myth of the day. Our culture believes in a rationality it cannot rationalize. This paradox is aptly described by the word *scientism*.

Manufacturing Illusions

The French thinker Paul Virilio makes a telling observation when he explores the etymological roots of the word *media*. It arises from the verb *to mediate,* a practice cultivated to perfection by Napoleon. Whenever the French army had overrun another country or province, its king or strongman was "mediated." This meant that the strongman was allowed to maintain possession of token insignia of his erstwhile power, such as a crown or other regalia. He was allowed to maintain the illusion of power, when in reality he was reduced to receiving and implementing the directives from the central government. He was mediated.

The word *mediate,* then, describes the process of rendering an individual powerless, albeit with the illusion of being in charge. This is what large segments of commercial media do. They mediate—in other words, render powerless—the public.

Virilio goes on to observe that commercial media, especially TV, lie shamelessly by omission and selection. An example can be found in the customary reports about medical breakthroughs, which typically appear on page three of the newspaper: the breakthrough is always by corporate pharmacology, is always a new, "promising" drug. By contrast, in order to read about other approaches to healing we have to venture past the mainstream media. Big media communicates a single philosophy: that corporate science and only corporate science will create solutions to health problems. This is the big strategic lie.

There are also tactical lies: studies favorable to a drug are published;

unfavorable ones are not. Sadly, this appears to be the rule, not the exception. A "system of illusions" is solidly in place and the real question is not whether or not these indefensible practices are a regrettable exception, but whether Pfizer is fundamentally different from Enron. If the purpose of a corporation is to mine or extract value for shareholders, then corporate pharmacology has made the lifestyle drugs such as Viagra or Tamoxifen—its tools to mine the human body—for shareholder value.

As deception has become an integral part of economic activity, it is vital that we examine the style and quality of the information we absorb for signs of misrepresentation or veracity.

Learning about Essential Oils Debunks Manufactured Illusions

When "swine flu" reared its head, the media machine did what it always does: it dramatized reporting of new cases alternating with the incessant mentioning of corporate antiviral drugs. The only concern seemed to be whether or not there were sufficient supplies to protect the most vulnerable demographics. That the efficacy of the mentioned drugs against H1N1 was apparently close to zero was not newsworthy. But it was so ineffective that the German weekly *Der Spiegel*—under no suspicion of having an anticorporate bias—called Tamiflu "modern man's amulet"!

Tamiflu and similar antivirals were developed to inhibit the enzyme neuraminidase (a transmembrane protein) of the influenza virus hull. This class of antivirals painfully illustrates the potential shortcomings of single target drugs. They may work under a very specific set of circumstances. But whenever the molecular target is slightly different—because it is a similar but not identical protein in a different virus, or because the targeted virus has mutated slightly—the monotarget drug is rendered ineffective. (See also "Recent Influenza Viruses: H1N1 Resistance" in chapter 10, page 144.)

This is the moment when we start to realize how resilient and life-supporting the nonselective mode of action of essential oils really is. Logic, reason, and available science support the contention that essential oils can be a most effective remedy to treat and especially prevent contracting the next influenza.

Personal experience is the best insurance for a degree of calm or at least realism and to be able to steer clear of panic or paranoia. The personal sense of relative safety—clearly there is never a 100 percent guarantee for total insulation from infection—arises from experience. This relative sense of safety comes with knowing how to use and apply essential oils and not feel threatened while doing so. It is like many things in life that require some time. When the next media blitz announces another viral epidemic, sensationalized or real, the reader will be best served by having already tried out ingesting some suitable essential oils. If we have never really utilized essential oils, trying them at the moment of the next threatened pandemic will only add to the sense of insecurity. But if we have already experienced antiviral essential oils and we are familiar with our body's response to them (particularly the nonoccurrence of any undesirable reaction), we will be much better equipped to deal with the situation effectively.

How Aromatherapy Really Progresses

In the field of aromatherapy it is informed lay individuals who often make the most relevant contributions, exploring and gradually adopting new approaches arising out of the recommendations of the pioneers.

A perfect example relates to the usefulness of Niaouli essential oil for protecting the skin from burns during radiation treatment. There was a small entry in the monograph section of the 1990 edition of *L'aromatherapie exactement,* proclaiming Niaouli essential oil (*Melaleuca quinquenervia viridiflora*) to be a "*protectrice cutané*" and then, modestly, in brackets, "*radioprotectrice.*" In addition the two protagonists, Pierre Franchomme and Daniel Pénoël, and probably other pioneers in the field, kept reiterating the radioprotectant properties of Niaouli essential oil. The information traveled through aromatherapy circles and at some point lay individuals tried it out. Ultimately Sylla Hanger's contribution at the 4th Aromatherapy Conference on the Therapeutic Uses of Essential Oils in 2000—"Use of Essential Oils to Counter Side Effects of Radiation during Cancer Treatments"—turned the sparse initial information into adaptable practical use.

A similar story lies behind the ascent of *Vitex agnus castus* essential oil. While the alcoholic extract of this plant has a long history in the herbal medicine of many societies, the essential oil had not really been a factor. At a phytotherapy conference in Munich, Dutch researcher J. H.

Zwaving, who soon after published results about research into the activity of *Vitex agnus castus*,[8] told aromatherapist Monika Haas he believed that the active components of the tincture of *Vitex agnus castus* would be much more prominently present in the essential oil. He expected the essential oil to be significantly more effective than the tincture. This notion was clearly confirmed by Barbara Lucks' study *"Vitex agnus castus:* Explorations in Menopausal Balance," also published in the *Proceedings of the 4th Aromatherapy Conference on the Therapeutic Uses of Essential Oils,* 2000. Essential oil of *Vitex agnus castus* is today used by many in the aromatherapy community as a highly effective and safe agent to equilibrate progesterone and estrogen levels, significantly easing PMS and menopausal complaints.

ESSENTIAL OIL JOURNEY

Lavender Authenticity

Lavender essential oil can serve as an example for many aromatherapy phenomena. It also illustrates a not-so-pleasant fact: the degree to which adulterated essential oils permeate the market. In Provence, cultivations of population Lavender—also referred to as *Lavande fine* and "Fine Lavender"—are few and far between the endless stretches of Lavandin. As a matter of fact, Fine Lavender is currently only cultivated on the plateaus of Saignon and Lagarde d'Apt, as well as in some areas around Mont Ventoux.

French export data shows that approximately 250 tons of so-called Fine Lavender are exported annually. The statistics of the association of Lavender growers in Volx show that less than 20 tons are in fact distilled. Ironically, this glaring fraud is obvious to those who can read the gas chromatograms, ostensibly recorded to demonstrate purity. Generally neither local vendor nor customer can read the chromatogram, but both associate proof of authenticity with its sheer existence. In reality most Lavender chromatograms passed around in the marketplace prove adulteration.

Given that Lavender essential oil is reconstructed by artful mixing of its main components linalool and linalyl acetate with more artfully mixed Lavandins, concentrations of linalool and linalyl acetate are typically very high in reconstructed Lavender oils.

Following are some typical markers for authentic Fine Lavender.

- The sum of linalool plus linalyl acetate is never more than 80% in authentic Fine Lavender.
- The sum of cis and trans ocimenes (common monoterpene hydrocarbons) should at least be 9%.

- Lavadulyl acetate is a compound that is specifically telling, because it cannot be purchased inexpensively on the market, but is made by nature in Lavender essential oil. Its concentration should be at least 4.5% in Fine Lavender.
- Finally, the concentration of camphor should be below 0.5%.

For a detailed description of the different types of Lavender plants that are cultivated, as well as the resulting essential oils, see *Aroma* magazine.[9]

Lavender: Where Do the Hybrids Come From?

Prior to the World War I era, Lavender essential oil was produced almost exclusively from wild plants growing in the French and Italian Alps. Lavender was harvested from Cuneo in Italy to the famous village of Barrême on the French side of the Sea Alps. Given the extreme poverty of the soil in the higher elevations of Provence and the dire economic situation after WWI, the local farmers looked for a cash crop that could produce extra income. They found that cash crop in Lavender, which thrives at the higher elevations of Provence.

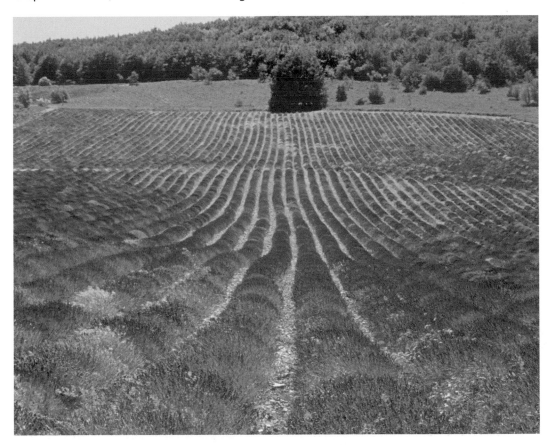

Population Lavender grown on the Plateau of Lagarde d'Apt

Today, most of the large cultivated areas of Provence are planted with different Lavandin hybrids, mostly *Grosso, Super, Sumian,* and *Abrialis*. Once *L. angustifolia* was cultivated between 1,800 and 2,400 feet, natural radiation carried seeds to lower lying areas. Spike Lavender (*Lavandula latifolia*) grows abundantly in the coastal areas of southern France, radiating upward to the mid-elevations where it meets *L. angustifolia*. On hillside prairie land in Provence, at about 1,400 to 1,800 feet, Fine Lavender, Spike, and their hybrid can be detected growing side by side in the wild. In the 1930s enterprising growers quickly found out that the essential oil content of the hybrid plants was substantially higher than that of *L. angustifolia*. A certain M. Grosso proceeded to clone a hybrid plant he found particularly attractive. The massive expanses of Lavandin Grosso seen in Provence today all go back to that one plant!

The largest area of more or less continuous Lavandin cultivation is the plateau of Valensole where blue stretches from horizon to horizon. The essential oils are very useful when organic, but do reflect the human intention for high yield and robust fragrance.

Provence: Perpetual Allure

Some locations in Provence have become familiar far beyond the actual region. Most famous of course are the attractions along the coast from Monaco and Grasse to Nice, St. Tropez, Toulon, and Marseille. But inland sensations are just as plentiful. Arguably more people will remember the image of the Abbey de Senanque than its name.

One of those Provencal sites, conveying romance and associations of gentle floral breezes, lives on in the Lavender trade. Many vendors still offer a Lavender provenance named after the village of Barrême, a little village on the slopes of the Alps in the Department Alpes-de-Haute-Provence, implying a particular fine high Alpine quality. However, the casual traveler passing through Barrême will be surprised not to find a single Lavender plant there, let alone the massive plant inventory needed to support the barrels of Lavender sold under that designation. Harvesting wild Lavender in difficult high Alpine terrain is no longer cost effective. It stopped a hundred years ago. While it is doubtful there is any production of Lavender in the higher French Alps, there are some small nostalgic operations on the Italian side in the surroundings of Cuneo.

Feeling an Essential Oil

Some aromatherapy authors say that immersion in essential oils taught them much more than learning their specific therapeutic applications. These authors claim that essential oils can teach broad lessons about health and even life in general. In other words, engaging with essential oils is presented as an avenue to building awareness about physiological and emo-

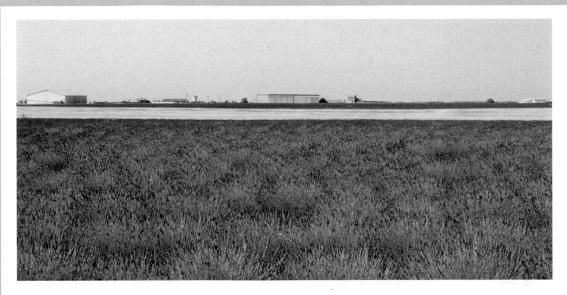

The Plateau de Valensole, approximately 12 miles wide by 24 miles long,
is arguably the largest expanse cultivated entirely in blue.

tional aspects of life that are otherwise often overlooked. This exercise explores awareness-building with essential oils.

To make this exercise casual and free of concerns about safety or even toxicity, the most benign and friendly essential oil is at its center. Lavender essential oil is the aromatherapy staple number one. Essential oils from hybrids, clones, and populations are readily available and serve well to experience some basic aromatherapy and essential oil concepts.

First, select a grooming activity that you enjoy on a daily basis. Showers are a good candidate, but using a body oil to nourish the skin is also a good option. It should be something that you do more or less every day, in which you can incorporate the topical use of essential oils.

Begin with organic Lavandin super oil. During your shower, put a specific amount, let's say 5 to 10 drops, into your hand and evenly distribute it on your feet, over and behind your knees, and upward over your torso all the way to your underarm area and neck.

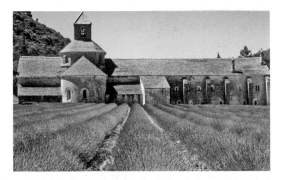

The image of the Abbey de Senanque has become a visual term for the travel industry, symbolizing everything pertaining to Provence.

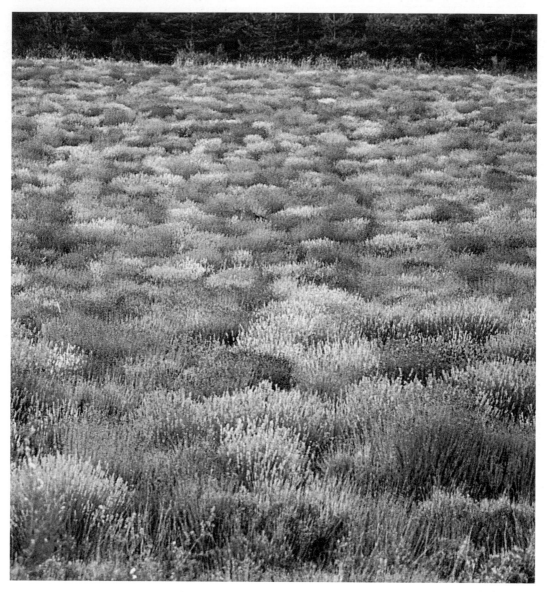

Fields of population Lavender are easily distinguished from the uniformity of hybrids and clones such as Maillette. The individual plants display wildly varying colors, reflecting sexual reproduction.

This procedure should be repeated for five days with the same oil. You will slowly develop an awareness of the subtle changes in mood and feeling that the oil precipitates. Do not expect any major revelations, but be sensitive to little flashes of well-being.

After five days of using Lavandin, switch to a clonal *Lavandula angustifolia* such as organic Maillette or Matheronne. Again, use this oil for some days. After this second trial you will have a

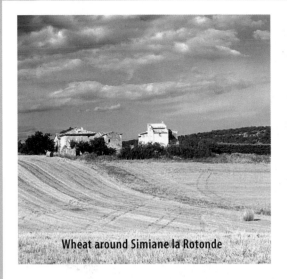
Wheat around Simiane la Rotonde

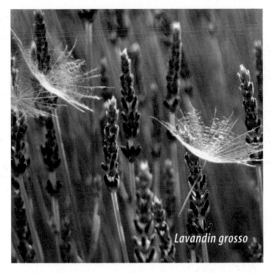
Lavandin grosso

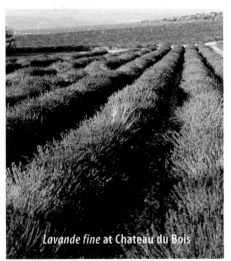
Lavande fine **at Chateau du Bois**

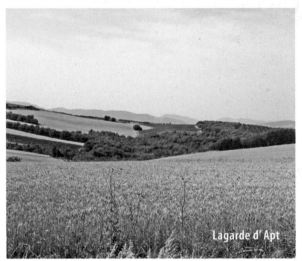
Lagarde d' Apt

Scenes from Haute Provence

fairly clear idea about the difference between the feel of the hybrid and the feel of the clonal Lavender.

In the third segment of the experiment, use population Lavender in exactly the same fashion as the two other oils. You will quickly become aware of the much softer quality of the population Lavender and how a lesser fragrance intensity goes along with increased complexity and elegance.

Before you know it you will have viscerally acquired the distinctions between hybrid, clonal, and population Lavenders.

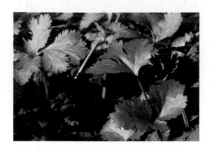

SIX

AROMATHERAPY CONNECTS WITH DIVERSE TRADITIONS

The exclusive reign of rational thought and science has led to the complete blindness of modern humanity for otherworldly beings.

WOLF-DIETER STORL

BACKGROUND INFORMATION

Grasse Symposium on Aromatherapy and Medicinal Plants

The Grasse Symposium has become the primary venue for French-style medical aromatherapy.

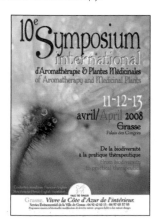

As of the early twenty-first century, many diverse approaches have been projected onto aromatherapy. The almost mythical writings of the Austrian-born biochemist Marguerite Maury, the contributions of French aromatherapy driven by science and medicine, the slightly neo-colonial attitudes of some British writers, and the esoteric texts of some German authors are all variations on the theme of how to use essential oils. The authors generally aspire to heal or treat disease, prevent premature aging, or attain states of higher consciousness. In this chapter we take a look at how some of these influences have manifested and how they offer varying approaches for many different situations in life.

Drawing from diverse systems of therapeutic reasoning is a defining strength of aromatherapy. As humans observed how they reacted to plant medicines, their view was invariably colored by their respective culture. But the object of observation—the unfolding biological mechanisms—are always the same. There are different methods of choosing essential oils for a specific condition. They differ by approaching the power of secondary plant metabolites from different angles, but they share the goal of understanding plant-human interaction.

French-Style Medical Aromatherapy

The connection between perfume plants and humans seems to be a timeless reality in the south of France. Geographic and climatic conditions favor the proliferation of many perfume plants—we need only think of the amazing fragrance of *Rosa gallica*. Fragrant plants were processed in the region as early as the eleventh century to improve the odor of leather produced in the local tanneries.

There is then a straight line from fragrancing leather to the Renaissance courts to the glorious age of Grasse as the perfume capital of the world. One must assume that the medicinal qualities of the local flora, including the perfume plants, were more or less known to the population throughout that time.

Then—beginning in the second half of the nineteenth century—these qualities were described in the language of modern science and chemistry. It is most fascinating to scan the references in Gattefossé's original book, published in 1937.

Even before the turn of the century there were publications about the antibacterial properties of many plant essential oils. As chemistry developed, chemists Charabot and Dupont began classifying the components of essential oils. This probably marks the very first manifestations of modern aromatherapy. Gattefossé elaborated on these classifications and coined the term "aromatherapy." This led directly to the evolution of the theoretical framework of the Valnet and Belaiche school of thought into what is now called "French-style aromatherapy."

Original French-style aromatherapy focused on the treatment of infections. It was similar to allopathic medicine in its intent to attack the pathogen. It was different in that it used natural agents instead of sulfonamides or antibiotics. In the French perspective, aromatherapy is a medical method to treat disease with essential oils, practiced and popularized by physicians. This scientific and professional approach was transformed into a modality accessible to the public in Robert Tisserand's groundbreaking book *The Art of Aromatherapy*.

Germ Theory and French-Style Aromatherapy

Nineteenth-century chemist and microbiologist Louis Pasteur discovered that bacteria can be the cause of infectious disease. To this day, especially in American culture, the concept of bacteria is that of the evil

Jean Valnet

Jean Valnet's book *Aromathérapie* (English title *The Practice of Aromatherapy*) was first published in 1964. It revived the idea of medicinal use of essential oils at a critical time when synthetic antimicrobial drugs such as sulfonamides and antibiotics seemed to have all but won the battle for medical dominance.

Valnet cultivated the popular knowledge about aromatic plants, which is so solidly rooted in the traditions of the south of France. His writings are clearly influenced by his scientific predecessors such as Charabot, Dupont, and Gattefossé but also by traditional wisdom as represented by Mességué. Valnet's work clearly created renewed respect for essential oils in the French medical establishment in ways never repeated in the anglophonic societies.

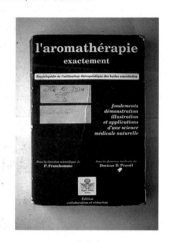

pathogen at the root of all disease. It is true that bacterial pathogens can be a dangerous reality, but it is also true that the single-minded blaming of bacteria for everything that ails us is a unique feature of Western medicine.

This self-destructive bacteriophobia is a vivid example of the staying power of the static illusions we seem to cherish. Ironically even Pasteur realized late in life that the singular focus on bacterial pathogens as the cause of disease was misleading. His famous statement was "The terrain is everything and the bacterium is nothing." Bacteria only survive in specific environments and need specific conditions to reproduce. This is only rarely mentioned. The easy availability of antibiotics leads to lax prevention! The continued rule of germ theory is probably not so much due to the validity of the assumption but rather a reflection of corporate pharmacology's stakes in maintaining this perception.

From a contemporary holistic angle, it appears that bacterial infection happens when the immune system is weakened and gives in to a known pathogen *or* when our body is subjected to an unknown pathogen and the immune system has yet to generate the appropriate antibodies. Realistically, some bacterial infections could be seen as a consequence of underlying weaknesses whereas others are due to the immune system being surprised by unfamiliar pathogens.

Given that in the early twenty-first century large segments of the population are entirely dependent on industrial antibiotics, the work of French physicians to develop effective essential oil treatments for bacterial infections appears highly prescient.

Classic French Three-Step Strategy for Infection Treatment

In French aromatherapy, infection treatment is generally styled according to a three-step strategy originally developed by Paul Belaiche in the late 1970s:

1. Supporting the elimination of toxins (e.g. cleansing the mucous membranes of pus)
2. Eliminating residual pathogens
3. Supporting convalescence

Belaiche published a large body of in vitro studies and actual clinical results showing the successful treatment of a broad range of infectious diseases using essential oils. In one form or another this three-step strategy has remained at the core of French aromatherapy.

Protocols based on this three-step strategy were developed by French physicians in the late 1970s, thereby remaining a specialty of conventional medicine inside France. This development was followed by the mainstream success of aromatherapy in the UK, where becoming an aromatherapist blossomed into a bona fide vocational concept.

The Structure Effect Model

Meanwhile French pioneers like Pierre Franchomme began to popularize a system that rationalized essential oil properties and facilitated their selection process. The structure effect model fleshes out the analytical basis of the three-step strategy. It contends that basic physiological and pharmacological properties are associated with the different types of terpenoid molecules present in essential oils. "Structure effect" was a bold design, which for the first time connected molecular and physical properties of essential oil components with their physiological activity. It provided the possibilities for a distinct formalism in assigning essential oils to disease conditions they could positively affect.

This opened up an extensive playground for subsequent authors, who found ample possibilities to insert their own modifications and twists. I published *Advanced Aromatherapy,* which explained the synergistic properties of some fifty essential oils by means of the Structure and Energy map (another name for the Structure Effect Diagram). In Germany, a book was published that attempted to unify the physical with the emotional and esoteric! Despite the disdain by the influential *International Journal of Aromatherapy* (IJA), which dismissively dubbed the system "functional group theory," it made inroads in British aromatherapy: based on "structure effect," a computerized mixing guide that allows the user to determine the best blend for a desired action with a mouse-click was published in the UK.[1]

British-Style Aromatherapy

Beginning in the 1980s, British-style aromatherapy made a big splash. Many books were published that told the public the oils to use and the oils to avoid. In retrospect, it can be said that these books were long

Plant Medicine: Simple and Available

Eighty percent of the world population lives outside the availability of Western medicine. The treatment methods and medications of this huge majority are often considered inferior to those of Western medicine. That may be true when measured by the tests of corporate pharmacology, but we can almost expect that it would enforce its own bias.

When a happy and healthy life is the measure, simple means all of a sudden don't look so bad.

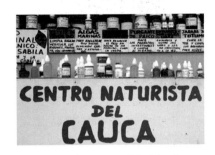

Outdoor pharmacy in Cali, Colombia

Aromatherapy Connects with Diverse Traditions

Structure Effect Diagrams

The illustration shows a typical representation of the structure effect diagram. The placement of the circles or ovals in the different quadrants reflects the electropositive (top) or electronegative (bottom) as well as the polar (left) or nonpolar (right) character of the main constituents of a given oil. The aldehydes components of Melissa accordingly are of electronegative and polar character, the terpenes of Lemon are electropositive and nonpolar. Listed below are the chemical families, which determine to a large degree the overall character of the oils represented in the diagram:

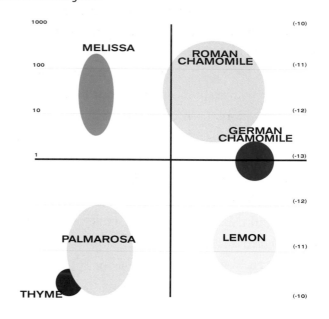

Melissa: citral, aldehydes

Roman Chamomile: esters

German Chamomile: sesquiterpene hydrocarbons

Lemon: monoterpene hydrocarbons

Palmarosa: terpene alcohols

Thyme: monoterpenoid phenols

on authoritative attitude and short on actual insight. Treatment suggestions for specific conditions were typically given ex cathedra. Rarely was there a discernible attempt to articulate an actual rationale as to why essential oils have physiological activity. Parallel to a growing number of enthusiastic authors, some self-appointed guardians of the scientific grail emerged, complaining about the lack of "science." Given that even then science had already morphed into an adjunct of the economic interest of large corporations, the alignment of these critics with fragrance industry research to this day appears rather ludicrous.

Chinese Medical Aromatherapy

The theoretical framework of Chinese medicine provides an alternative way to approach the therapeutic potential of essential oils. Like Chinese herbal mixtures, essential oils consist of partly more- and partly less-effective components. Like Chinese herbal mixtures, essential oils appear to be of a composition that minimizes side effects and optimizes efficacy.

Taoist master Jeffrey Yuen has pioneered a form of aromatherapy best referred to as "Chinese medical aromatherapy." He applies the perspective of classical Chinese medicine to the use of essential oils. Hence a few examples of Yuen's language and contentions shall be given, as they have an extraordinary capacity to empower the individual searching for healing strategies.

Note of Caution: I do not in any way claim to be an expert in classical Chinese medicine. The following basic ideas have been taken from the presentations of Jeffrey Yuen and are intended to stimulate the reader to explore this fascinating field at greater depth.

Paradigm of Chinese Medicine

Classical Chinese medicine is based on the philosophical framework of Taoism and consequently approaches healing with a broader outlook than Western medicine. According to Yuen, Chinese medicine operates from the fundamental notion that there are "preconditions of life," which need to be met for healthy living. Those preconditions are:

Survival: access to nutrition and being able to fulfill fundamental physiological needs

Interaction: typically interactions with other humans, often evolving into the search for meaning

Differentiation: adjustment or refinement of our worldview and habits as we go through life

Aromatherapy can play significant roles in meeting the requirements of all three preconditions. For example, essential oils can aid in survival by treating infections. They can support interaction by making readjustments of our place in life and society easier. Issues of interaction most often arise for individuals in their thirties and forties in the shape of conditions resulting from excess stress.

While relevant for survival and interaction, essential oils are uniquely suited to help when we are challenged to change our outlook or worldview, when we need to differentiate. Connecting with essential oils can become a key element to facilitate these changes.

When it comes to treating disease, Yuen emphasizes the difference between Western and Chinese approaches. Chinese medicine does not treat diseases but rather individual patients. It is perfectly normal for Chinese medicine to treat two individuals differently, despite the fact

CONTRIBUTORS TO AROMATHERAPY

Jeffrey Yuen

In an emerging trend in alternative medical communities, most notably in New York and California, aromatherapy has turned to the interface of Chinese medicine and essential oils. This movement was more or less single-handedly pioneered by Taoist Master Jeffrey Yuen.

Mr. Yuen articulates the healing properties of essential oils based on the philosophical concepts of Chinese medicine. His aim is not so much to match specific symptoms with specific remedies but instead to empower the individual (therapist) to apply the concepts of Chinese medicine to recognize essential oil properties relevant for a specific patient.

BACKGROUND INFORMATION

Japanese Kampo

The approach of Kampo medicine in Japan is similar to that of traditional Chinese medicine's herbal mixtures, where analysis of the contribution of single components to the effectiveness of the complete synergy is not of primary interest, but rather the effect of the whole combination of herbs.[2]

Aromatherapy Connects with Diverse Traditions

Aromatics in Chinese Medicine

Essential oils are mentioned in the first herbal of Chinese medicine, *Shen Nong Ben Cao,* written in the second century CE. It classifies plants as useful in the categories of prevention, restoration, and treatment. Commentaries on the *Ben Cao* specify parts of plants such as leaves and stems as well as their *jing* (essence), which corresponds to our understanding of essential oil. In the sixteenth century the famous herbal *Ben Cao Gang Mu,* by Li Shihzhen, details the therapeutic use of a number of essential oils, including Ginger, Camphor, and Rose.

that their Western diagnosis is the same. Whereas Western medicine assumes disease symptoms are caused by a pathogen, Yuen contends that disease symptoms often are not primarily caused by the original pathogen, but instead represent the response of the body trying to correct imbalances or blockages caused by the pathogen. In Yuen's perspective the most promising course of action is to remedy the imbalance rather than simply counteracting a symptom.

Main Characteristics of Plant Essential Oils

From the perspective of traditional Chinese medicine (TCM), three main characteristics of plant essential oils determine their therapeutic application: variability, sensory impact, and resonance with *yuan qi,* or the "original" form of the body's vital energy. (For more about the role of the different aspects of *qi,* vital energy, in traditional Chinese medicine, refer to the side panel on page 99, "The Three Layers of Qi.")

1. Variability

The Western and the Chinese approach both recognize that essential oils of identical species originating from different populations may vary in their fragrance or in their qualities. This qualitative variability is a consequence of the plant's state in its life cycle, its growing conditions, and the way the plant organism expresses itself. The difference arises in how this variability is valued. In Western pharmacology variation is an impediment to a constant product quality. In the Chinese perspective qualitative variability is a key factor in the therapeutic efficacy of essential oils. This is congruent with the recognition of evolutionary biology that constant variation of composition is an important factor preventing microorganisms from developing resistance to essential oils.

2. Sensory Impact

Eastern and Western philosophical views and Western scientific thought all agree that our senses provide us—literally and figuratively—with our "worldview," or with what we consider to be real.

According to Chinese medicine, the sensory organs are situated in the sphere of and correlate with *wei qi* (defensive vital energy). As a consequence, essential oils modify the way our sensory organs process information. As the sensory organs change, so does the information delivered to the brain and, ultimately, the way we see the world. (See

"John Eccles on the Construction of Reality" sidebar, page 116.) This change is often a most important step in the healing process. This is especially true if we accept that the consciousness leading into disease cannot be the one leading out of it. A change in consciousness is seen as the most effective way to discontinue pathological patterns at the root of disease. Yuen contends that aromatherapy helps individuals to arrive at necessary behavioral changes, hence he refers to aromatherapy as a self-differentiating modality.

3. Resonance with Yuan Qi

In Chinese herbal medicine, the extracted essence represents the basic design element of the plant or an expression of the script that directs all of its energetic processes, ranging from growth to decline. In this respect, essential oils relate first and foremost with yuan qi. Taoist cultivators even expand the idea of the plant's aromatic essence to include the liberation of its soul. (In a Western sense yuan qi or original qi corresponds to the hormones, marrow, and sexual fluids, respectively growth factors, immunity, and the basis for procreation.)

Chinese medicine contends that essential oils interact with yuan/original qi to influence disease processes where the constitution or the genetic program have been injured or taxed by a pathogen. Interestingly this is fully in line with Western research that demonstrates the antitumor effects of essential oils (see chapter 13).

The Interaction of Essential Oils with Wei Qi and Ying Qi

Essential oils are also active on the planes of wei qi and ying qi. Essential oil resonance with wei qi results in increased adaptability to adverse environmental conditions and manifests in the effectiveness of essential oils against viral, bacterial, and fungal pathogens. Essential oils can also help

Practical Applications of Essential Oils

In China essential oils are generally applied either externally as ointments or creams or internally, added to herbal preparations shortly before consumption. Such applications are aimed at nourishing the "blood" and the endocrine system. Another classic application of essential oils in Chinese medicine, mainly from the yuan qi perspective, is to "glue wounds," which is directed at chronic and nonhealing ulcers.

Aromatherapy Connects with
Diverse Traditions

As we have seen, the Western view of medicine focuses on the molecular structures of drugs. The typical sequence of medical development starts with a molecule synthesized in the lab, or alternatively derived from an unknown plant of the Amazon jungle, followed by a test for efficacy. In Western drug research the molecule comes first and physiological functionality is accepted as a random occurrence.

The classical Chinese view is quite different. It is not concerned with molecular composition but almost exclusively with function. Like Ayurveda, traditional Indian medicine, it is based on the observation of plant-human interactions over a long period of time. As a result, the Chinese medical system has empirically recognized the healing properties of many plants without making any statement about active ingredients or molecular structures. To articulate this with the terminology of modern biology, it has observed the properties arising at the level of organization of the whole plant organism.

to build blood or stimulate metabolic turnover and improve elimination of metabolic waste and xenochemicals.

The Therapeutic Spectrum of Chinese Medical Aromatherapy

Essential oils are uniquely appropriate to address conditions in which the integrity of the genetic program has been compromised. This includes civilization diseases such as asthma, neurodermatitis, fibromyalgia, ulcerative colitis, chronic fatigue syndrome, systemic candidiasis, and other cases of systemic dysbiosis. Recent studies confirm that monoterpene and sesquiterpene components of essential oils prevent carcinogenesis. For the skilled acupuncturist, applying essential oils in minute quantities to acupoints that relate to jing essence has been found to be an effective contribution in addressing the mentioned conditions.

Connecting Essential Oils and the Five Elements

Choosing essential oils for an individual according to the five element theory will enhance the individual's adaptive abilities toward ecological/environmental/climatic factors, thus making possible the reduction or elimination of the use of antibiotics. From the Chinese medical perspective, improved immunity against pathogens is a consequence of the uninhibited flow of wei qi but also that of strengthened identity through yuan qi resonance.

FIVE ELEMENTS AND ESSENTIAL OILS

Wood Excess: Chamomile, Lavender, Lemon, Spikenard

Wood Deficiency: Carrot Seed, Chamomile, Rose, Vetiver

Fire Excess: Lemon Verbena, Sweet Marjoram, Neroli, Orange, Valerian

Fire Deficiency: Frankincense, Sage, Sandalwood

Earth Excess: Cardamom, Patchouli, Petitgrain

Earth Deficiency: Caraway, Coriander

Metal Excess: Citronella, Eucalyptus, Myrtle, Ravintsara

Metal Deficiency: Fir, Hyssop linalool, Niaouli, Pine, Thyme linalool

Water Excess: Cedarwood, Juniper

Water Deficiency: Basil, Clary Sage, Geranium

Interaction of Plants and Humans in Asia

Jeffrey Yuen has pioneered the synthesis of aromatherapy and a Chinese medical perspective. Yuen's guidelines are a most useful recognition of the multiple properties of essential oils. Following are some examples of Yuen's characterizations, juxtaposed with some key properties as listed in *L'aromatherapie exactement*. This compilation is not intended to be a guide to using essential oils in a TCM (traditional Chinese medicine) fashion. Instead it is meant as another demonstration of how plant-human interaction is a constant of human life. The Chinese indications listed with each oil are excerpted from

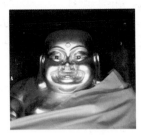

Buddha in Doi Suthep,
Chiang Mai

Materia Medica of Essential Oils (Based on a Chinese Medical Perspective) by Jeffrey Yuen.[3]

Anethum graveolens
Mucolytic, stimulates bile

(1) Descends lung qi to release coughing
(2) Resolves food stasis, bile secretion, and lactation

Angelica archangelica
Anxiety, abdominal cramps

(1) Tonifies lung and spleen qi, stimulates appetite
(2) Nourishes blood and calms the shen (spirit)
(3) Opens the diaphragm to expel phlegm
(4) Regulates liver overaction on spleen and stomach

Anthemis nobilis
Nervous shock

(1) Regulates liver qi and liver fire
(2) Nourishes liver blood and subdues wind
(3) Calms shen: irritability, restlessness, insomnia

Apium graveolens
Drains the liver

(1) Regulates liver to consolidate yin
(2) Drains dampness and expels wind-damp bi (obstruction)
(3) Clears fire toxins
(4) Descends stomach qi, bloating, belching, vomiting

Artemisia dracunculus
Spasmolytic, antiviral, PMS

(1) Regulates stomach qi, vomiting, hiccups
(2) Promotes menstruation

Boswellia carterii
Depression

(1) Alleviates anxiety and depression
(2) Relieves stomach ulcers, fibrocystic breast and kidneys
(3) Reduces swelling and treats nonhealing wounds
(4) Relaxes the diaphragm to promote circulation of lung qi and deep breathing (asthma, bronchitis)
(5) Invigorates the blood and calms the shen (spirit)

Cananga odorata
Antidiabetic, tachycardia, sexual tonic

(1) Clears heat in the blood, high blood pressure
(2) Calms the shen, anger, frustration, fear, jealousy
(3) Arouses kidney essence, useful for impotence

Cinnamomum zeylanicum
Tropical infections

(1) Warms the middle and lower heater to expel cold
(2) Invigorates blood to promote menstruation
(3) Strengthens ming-men (energetic center storing yuan qi) fire

Cistus ladaniferus
Antiviral, fights scarlet fever, whooping cough

(1) Regulates liver overacting on the spleen
(2) Stops bleeding
(3) Astringes

Citrus auranthium leaves
Nervous depression, arterial hypertension

(1) Regulates qi in the chest and epigastrium
(2) Calms the shen
(3) Strengthens memory by transforming dampness

Citrus reticula
Overexcitement

(1) Strengthens spleen's transformation
(2) Descends stomach qi
(3) Calms shen: insomnia
(4) Subdues interior wind: epilepsy, spasms

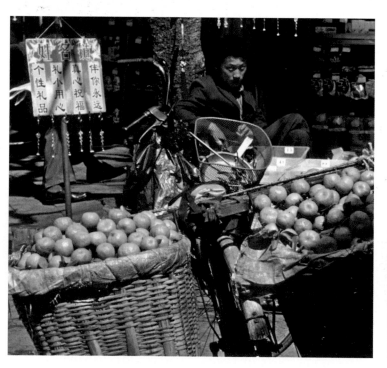

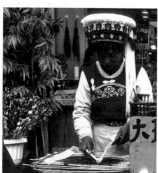

Bird and Flower Market, Kunming. Symbolism accompanies the celebration of the Chinese New Year: oranges represent wealth and tangerines good luck.

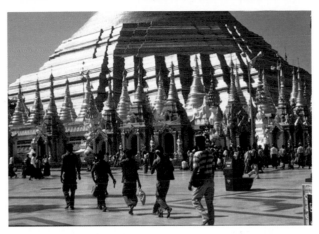

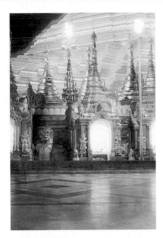

As the setting sun casts its last rays on the soft orange dome of the great Shwedogon Paya, one feels the magic in the air. In the heat of the day, the stupa glitters bright gold. It can be quiet and contemplative or colorful and raucous. The Golden Dragon is the essence of Myanmar, a place that never fails to enchant.

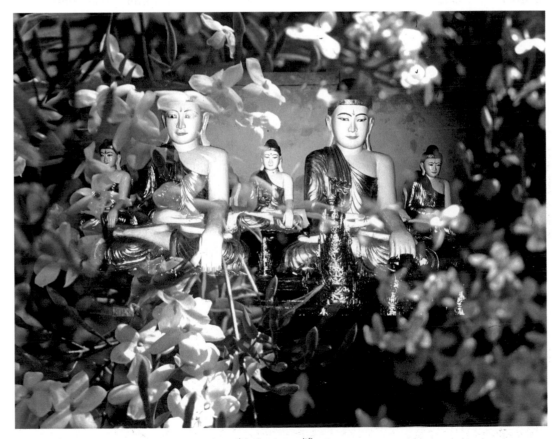

Jasminum grandiflorum

Citrus sinensis
Anxiety

(1) Releases wind-heat with fever, chills, cough
(2) Clears heart fire, arrhythmia, insomnia, hypertension
(3) Descends stomach qi to promote peristalsis

Commiphora molmol
Antiviral, anti-inflammative

(1) Clears lung and stomach heat, thick yellow sputum coughing, gum swellings, toothache, hyperthyroidism
(2) Strengthens the spleen, flatulence, loss of appetite
(3) Invigorates the blood for bruises and varicose veins
(4) Promotes wound healing

Coriandrum sativum
Asthenia, arthrosis

(1) Releases exterior cold and dampness
(2) Transforms dampness and expels bi-obstruction
(3) Tonifies spleen qi

Cupressus sempervirens
Lymph, vein, and prostate decongestant

(1) Transforms dampness and clears lung heat
(2) Astringes fluid discharge
(3) Ascends spleen qi for prolapse
(4) Assists the kidney in grasping lung qi

Cymbopogon martinii
Urogenital infections, antiviral

(1) Releases wind-heat
(2) Regulates liver qi and clears damp-heat fire toxins

Cymbopogon nardus
Arthritis

(1) Clears heat in the wei level and repels pestilent qi

Daucus carota
Detoxifies liver and kidney, thyroid imbalance, eczema

(1) Nourishes liver blood
(2) Regulates liver overaction on the spleen

Hyssopus decumbens
Antiviral, nervous depression

(1) Clears lung heat

Inula graveolens
Hypertension, mucolytic

(1) Clears chronic lung heat
(2) Descends qi to calm rebellion and expel phlegm

Juniperus communis
Analgesic

(1) Expels wind-damp-cold bi-obstruction
(2) Drains damp-cold
(3) Promotes menstruation

Lippia citriodora
Anti-inflammative, sedative,
Crohn's, diabetes, depression

(1) Clears liver and heart fire: restlessness, anxiety, stress
(2) Regulates liver overacting on the stomach resulting
in nausea, vomiting, colic, epigastric burning,
foul breath

Litsea citrata
Nervous depression

(1) Tonifies spleen and kidney yang
(2) Expel wind-damp bi-obstruction
(3) Releases wind-cold with underlying deficiency
(4) Invigorates qi and blood in the lower abdomen

Majorana hortensis
Parasympathotonic, arthritis,
arthrosis

(1) Descends liver yang ascension and clears liver fire
(2) Releases wind-heat and wind-damp-hot bi-obstruction
(3) Alleviates cough, whooping cough, expels phlegm
(4) Descends stomach qi to promote peristalsis

Matricaria recutita
Decongestant, eczema

(1) Regulates liver qi, especially in the uterus
(2) Clears liver fire and subdues liver wind
(3) Harmonizes liver and its overacting on spleen/stomach
(4) Calms the shen (the hun, the spirit of wood)

Myrtus communis
Prostate decongestant,
hypothyroidism

(1) Clears lung heat and heat in the upper orifices
(2) Astringes leakage of qi and blood (e.g. sweating,
bleeding, hemorrhoids)

Nardostachys jatamansi
Psoriasis

(1) Clears heart fire palpitations, agitation, hysteria
(2) Subdues liver wind, headaches, seizures, facial ticks

Ocimum basilicum
Relaxant, reduces
sympathicus tonus

(1) Decongest veins and prostate, hepatitis, arthritis, MS,
tropical virus infections
(2) Descends stomach qi
(3) Resolves food stasis
(4) Tonifies kidney yang to drain dampness in the lower
heater

Pelargonium asperum
Tonifies lymph and veins,
pancreatic insufficiency,
arthritis, anxiety, hemorrhoids

(1) Nourishes kidney yin and establishes kidney heart
communication, calms the shen
(2) Regulates liver qi, PMS, fibrocystic breast, jaundice
(3) Descends stomach qi for food stasis
(4) Astringes fluid and blood loss in the lower heater

Picea mariana Eczema, prostate inflammation, asthenia, hypothyroidism	(1) Descends lung qi to the kidneys, coughing, asthma (2) Warms kidney yang (3) Expels wind-cold bi (obstruction)
Pinus sylvestris Asthenia, high blood pressure, diabetes, uterine and ovarian decongestant, asthma, arthritis, allergies	(1) Descends lung qi to kidneys, coughing, wheezing (2) Warms kidney yang for impotence (3) Transforms cold phlegm and expels wind-damp-cold bi-obstruction
Piper nigrum Rheumatism, asthenia	(1) Releases wind-cold with cold phlegm in the lungs (2) Warms the stomach to expel cold
Pogostemon cablin Vein tonic	(1) Releases the exterior and expels dampness (2) Harmonizes the middle heater, treats vomiting, nausea, lethargy, hemorrhoids, varicose veins, diarrhea (3) Transforms dampness (water retention) (4) Releases pent-up emotions
Salvia officinalis Herpes genitalis, condyloma, HPV	(1) Clears stomach fire, fever, sweat, sore throat, toothache, frontal headaches, mouth/gum ulcers, thrush, bad breath (2) Nourishes yin deficiency, amenorrhea, treats menopausal hot flashes, anxiety, insomnia, night sweat, false libido, dysmenorrhea (3) promotes bile production (e.g., damp-heat) (4) Breaks up fire toxins and phlegm stasis, fatty deposits, tumors
Satureja montana Hypotension (low blood pressure)	(1) Tonifies spleen qi and its production of blood (2) Expels intestinal worms (3) Transforms damp-phlegm

Aromatherapy Lifestyle

Something akin to an aromatherapy lifestyle has been articulated by U.S. aromatherapists, mainly originating in California. Essential oils are used to make everyday urban life healthier by providing easy means to manage crucial stress situations or by substituting for toxic household chemicals. Using essential oils outside the realm of therapeutic intervention is especially valuable, because it allows the curious layperson to develop a feel for essential oils, without the added concerns connected to self-medication.

The Pacific Institute of Aromatherapy (PIA) (see "Resources" at the back of the book for more information about PIA) sees itself as an integral part of this development. We have always advocated a style of aromatherapy that empowers the individual, the layperson, to utilize essential oils daily in simple but effective ways. Indeed, the frequent use of essential oils in itself brings back plant secondary metabolites that had been exorcised by our turn toward synthetic foods. Reintroducing those secondary metabolites with which the human organism has an intimate relation and that have been present in life forever dramatically improves the odds for healthy living. It reduces the occurrence of opportunistic illnesses (such as not contracting the flu when everyone else has it).

Perhaps even more importantly, many secondary metabolites work to maintain a balanced autonomic nervous system. By maintaining balance in the autonomic nervous system, an aromatherapy lifestyle

UNDERSTANDING AROMATHERAPY

Observing Function

Plants that proliferate successfully in arid conditions, at high altitude, or in bright sunlight need to prevent the loss of moisture. Such plants effectively seal themselves off. Their essential oils are a part of the biochemical design accomplishing this task. Nature-based traditions observe whether this transfers to the human body and maximize that capability for healing, such as in the case of the essential oil of *Cistus ladaniferus*, which is used to stop bleeding.

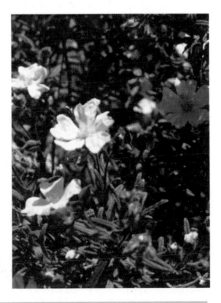

Rock Rose, *Cistus ladaniferus*, grows abundantly above the tree line in the Atlas Mountains of Morocco. It thrives in the relentless sun and manages to exist with minimal moisture.

Aromatherapy Connects with Diverse Traditions

prevents or delays the onset of more serious metabolic or degenerative diseases (even cancer) and allows an individual to live life as close as possible to the full potential of her or his constitution. For many essential oil users the incidence of serious disease is drastically reduced as a consequence of an aromatherapy lifestyle.

The more immediate understanding of the broad activity of secondary metabolites was integrated with the basic concepts of French-style aromatherapy by California aromatherapist Monika Haas of the PIA. She has developed a style of formulating that does not so much aim at specific symptoms, but, in keeping with the broad spectrum of activity of secondary metabolites, addresses broader health issues. In what represents a second generation of formulating in the French tradition, oils are blended to address a whole spectrum of symptoms associated with issues such as allergies, inflammation, insomnia, injuries, yeast overgrowth, pain, nervousness, or anxiety.

SEVEN

THE MYSTERY OF FRAGRANCE

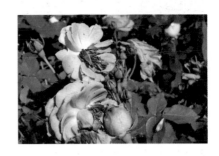

If you have two dirhams, take one to buy a loaf of bread for the stomach and take the other to buy hyacinths for the soul.

SPANISH MOORISH PROVERB

Spending half of one's assets on a fragrance reflects a view of life that does not find any counterpart in our materialistic world, where we are so used to characterizing everything by its monetary value. But, really, what price does the fragrance of a flower or the bouquet of a perfect old wine have? We have ample evidence that in the past plants had a place in human emotional and intellectual life no longer found in the digital age. For example, even a glance at *El Olfato,* a painting by Jan Brueghel

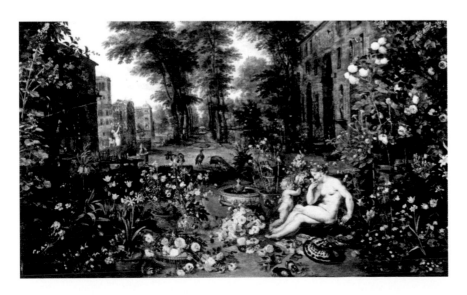

In *El Olfato*, Jan Brueghel the elder depicts nature and life as a grandiose, pleasant play for the senses. His allegories of the five senses are a fascinating study for everyone interested in symbolism.

109

the elder (1568–1625), confirms one of our basic notions about which fragrances we cherish: the fragrance of blossoming flowers in a garden and the fragrance of a living forest!

This painting dedicated to the sense of smell has apparently not been made the subject of a thorough analysis. Its open and veiled symbolism offer enchanting insight and should hold inspiration for the creation of aromatherapy synergies of one purpose or another.

In the following poem of Sor Juana Inés de la Cruz (1651–1695), Sonnet 147, excerpted from *The Golden Age—Poems of the Spanish Renaissance,* translated by Edith Grossman, we can also see evidence of the intimate relationship between a Renaissance mind and plant expression.

> *O rose divine, in gentle cultivation*
> *you are, with all your fragrant subtlety,*
> *tuition, purple-hued, to loveliness,*
> *snow-white instruction to the beautiful;*
> *intimation of a human structure,*
> *example of gentility in vain,*
> *in whose one being nature has united*
> *the joyful cradle and the mournful grave;*
> *how haughty in your pomp, presumptuous one,*
> *how proud when you disdain the threat of death,*
> *then, in a swoon and shriveling,*
> *you give a withered vision of a failing self;*
> *and so, with your wise death and foolish life,*
> *in living you deceive, dying you teach!*

Fragrance and Evolution

From the viewpoint of biology, fragrance perception and reactions to fragrance have an evolutionary component. Plant odorants have been present at every stage of biological evolution, interacting with receptor systems and initiating cascades of biological events. This evolutionary component is very much in evidence in our responses to familiar fragrances. Our reaction to a flowering garden is quite different from that to smoke or vinegar. There are, however, great difficulties in determining to what degree physiological responses to fragrance reflect cultural programming, hedonic responses, or congenital predisposition.[1] Nonetheless, a considerable body of knowledge has been accumulated in this area under the heading of the psychology of perfume.[2]

Pharmacology and Fragrance

In the Western perspective it is not disputed that fragrance can have dramatic impact on mood, emotion, and mating behavior, among other factors. Yet there has not been a systematic effort to employ fragrance for the physical betterment of a patient. In popular aromatherapy there are, however, some fairly well established fragrance effects, such as the effect of Neroli oil (*Citrus aurantium flores*) as an anxiolytic agent.

However, fragrance, sensory perception, and its value for healing do not resonate well with Western pharmacology. It appears that drug-development-oriented pharmacology would just as well not even deal with the phenomenon of fragrance, despite the fact that there have been studies on its fringes trying to objectify fragrance. There is an ironic twist to these efforts. Looking at the studies, one cannot help but sense that fragrance is something very threatening for the reductionist method, because it is impossible to measure. An odorant can be put through a gas chromatograph and its composition recorded. But then how can the associated fragrance be measured? Can it be expressed by saying "molecule A has five roses and three skunks on the open odor scale"? So it is not surprising that fragrance is met with a certain degree of disdain. It has the capacity to foul up otherwise neat pharmacological experiments.

In addition, fragrance thwarts double blind studies. The strong odor of essential oils is always an impediment as the essential oils will obviously have an odor and provisions have to be made to mask the odor so the "true" pharmacological effect of the oils can be observed.[3]

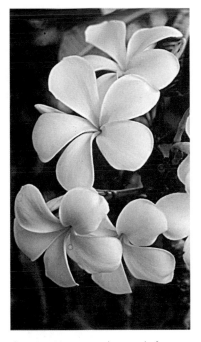

Frangipani is apparently named after the Italian Marquis do Frangipani. To this day, the *savoir vivre* (living well) celebrated on the Cote d'Azur as well as on the Riviera includes cherishing the flavors and fragrances of tropical and summer flowers and fruit. Many of the most celebrated scents of flowers remain elusive, because they are not stored in the plant or the flower like an essential oil. Instead they are continuously released by the plant metabolism. They are, so to speak, the breath of the living plant.

Essential Oils, the Senses, and Healing

Essential oils give rise to sensory impressions, first and foremost through their fragrance. However, we see their color, feel their liquid nature, or recognize sensations of heat or cooling when they are applied to the skin. We taste explosive layers of turpentine when we ingest them! As we have seen in chapter 2, essential oils generate many different physiological effects by modulating protein conformation.

Exploring Spain and Its Aromatic History

To live in the present and to enjoy beauty was characteristic of the Spanish Moors. The few remnants of their culture that have survived through time express this very clearly. In the late Middle Ages, with and because of ideologically veiled crusades against the infidels, the rich Moorish heritage was exorcised from the collective consciousness. Nonetheless, Western culture even today is inseparably influenced by all the advances of civilization that arose from Moors, Jews, and Christians living peacefully side-by-side in the glorious times of Al Andalus (the Arabic name for the Moorish parts of the Iberian peninsula, today partly identical with the Spanish region of Andalusia).

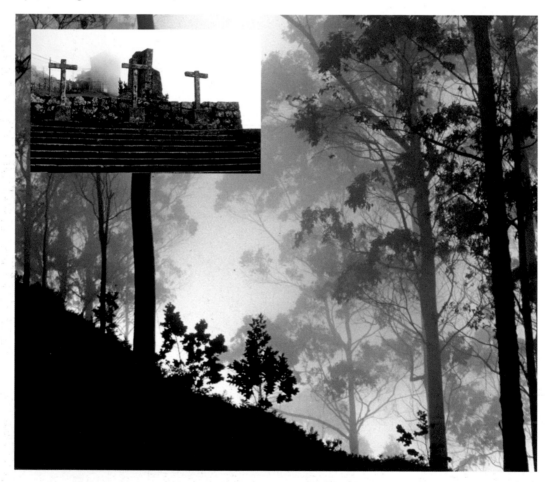

Eucalyptus lines the ascent to Monte Santa Tecla, the site of a Celtic settlement from around 3000 BCE, which apparently predated the Celtic influx to Ireland by more than 1,000 years. Bagpipes are the characteristic instrument of Galicia and the natives of this northernmost province of Spain proudly claim that Galicia indeed is the "Corazon Celta." Inset: Atop Monte Santa Tecla

Exploring the culture of medieval Cordoba and Al Andalus for its appreciation of sensuality and its tremendously rich repertoire of aromatics, spices, and foods very likely produces the most unexpected revelations.

An Andalusian Alphabet of Oriental Delights

Almond, Aloe, Ambra, Anise, Apricot, Balsam, Bay Laurel, Belladonna, Bergamot, Carob, Celery, Cinnamon, Clove, Couscous, Cocoa, Caper, Cardamom, Cassia, Coffee, Cumin, Curcuma, Date, Eggplant, Figs, Fennel, Frankincense, Garam Masala, Ginger, Grape, Honey, Jasmine, Lemon, Lime, Mace, Marjoram, Marzipan, Melon, Mint, Musk, Myrrh, Nutmeg, Olive, Orange, Oregano, Pepper, Peach, Pistachio, Pomegranate, Quince, Raisins, Rose, Rosemary, Saffron, Sandalwood, Sesame, Tamarind, Thyme, Violet, Wine

The Cathedral in Santiago de Compostela, one of Christianity's most revered pilgrimage destinations, boasts one of the largest Frankincense burners in the world.

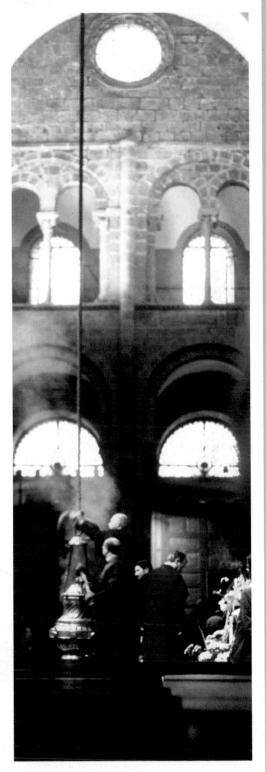

"Los Musicos" atop the Portica de Gloria in the Cathedral of Santiago de Compostela

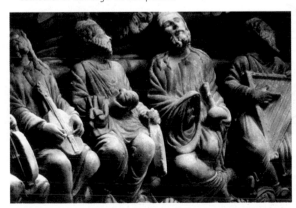

Citrus Tree of Many Uses

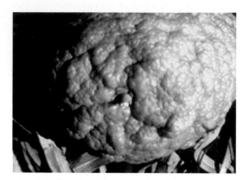

Bitter Orange or Seville Orange
(*Citrus aurantium*)

The citruses are small trees originating in oriental Asia, China, India, and Southeast Asia, belonging to the family of the *Rutaceae*. The word *orange* comes from the Arabic *narandj,* and it was in fact the Arabs who introduced not just the number zero but also the orange tree to Europe. Products made from citrus and essential oils being derived from rind, leaves, and petals point to an intense and beneficial relation between citrus and humans. Bitter Orange or Seville Orange (*Citrus aurantium*) is the perfect and often-cited example.

Citrus probably led to the first distillations in European history. The Arabs distilled Seville Oranges in the eleventh century for perfume. To this day the essential oil of the petals (Neroli) is one of the most precious essential oil specialties. It is generally tied to Old World traits such as long-term planning and steady ownership over generations. It takes years before oranges and petals can be harvested from Seville Orange trees. The trees in vital producing groves of Bitter Orange in the surroundings of Seville average an age of 100 years.

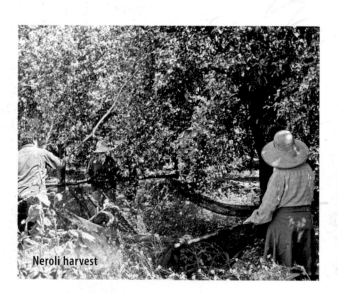

Neroli harvest

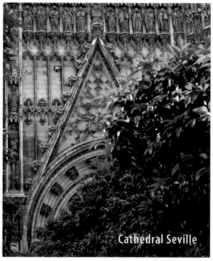

Cathedral Seville

Bitter Orange trees line the streets and parks of Seville. The extravagant cathedral of Seville is surrounded by squares planted with Bitter Orange as well. During Easter a thick layer of Bitter Orange fragrance provides the olfactory backdrop, as the city vibrates with the most intense celebrations.

The peel of the fruit is used for the famous and unique flavor of British marmalade. It is also used to make Bitter Orange Peel oil. Even though Bitter Orange Peel is generally described as sedative, it can also act as a gentle bitter tonic when used in low concentrations.

Petitgrain essential oil is distilled from the annual pruning of the leaves and tiny, very recently formed fruits, which are called *petit* (or "little") grains. This essence is appreciated in perfumery (as an indispensable element of eau de cologne) and aromatherapy alike. Petitgrain essential oil is nontoxic and can be used liberally in preparations used to address stress and imbalance of the autonomic nervous system.

Cold Pressing

Citrus peel oils—which are recovered by cold pressing—are fundamentally different from most other essential oils, which are steam distilled. Steam distillation limits the size of molecules traveling into in the essential oil, whereas cold pressing does not. Because of this, larger, photosensitizing coumarine molecules are generally present in citrus peel oils. The potential photosensitizing quality of these oils should be considered before using them topically.

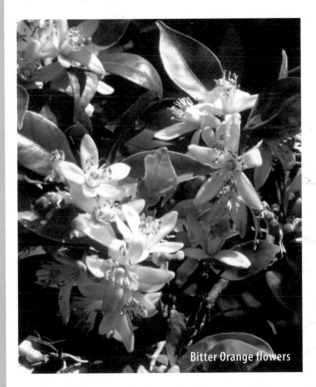
Bitter Orange flowers

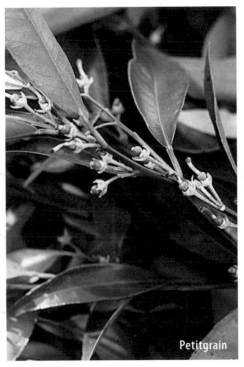
Petitgrain

Neroli (*Citrus aurantium*) essential oil is most notably produced in Spain, Tunisia, and Egypt. It displays the diversity of notions aromatherapy offers: its ability to ease anxiety speaks to our soul and its rejuvenating components unite the physical body with the desire for beauty.

Associations between Odor Qualities and the Five Elements

Wood: Herbaceous, Woody
Fire: Floral
Earth: Sweet, Fruity, Musty
Metal: Spicy, Sharp, Camphorous, Balsamic
Water: Moldy, Ocean, Salty

Sensory Impressions

Eastern and Western thought realize that we perceive the universe around us by means of our senses. What we believe to be real is ultimately the result of the sum of our sensory impressions and how we process and organize these enormous amounts of information.

John Eccles on the Construction of Reality

The idea that sensory perceptions construct our reality is neither an esoteric nor a lightweight tale. This notion is solidly established in Western (and Eastern) scientific and philosophical tradition. A key study to consult on this topic is Eccles' *The Evolution of the Brain*.[4]

Essential oils can also modulate the conformation of so-called G proteins, which are the signaling agents of the sensory organs. For example, as the retina perceives light, the resulting impression is transmitted to the brain. G proteins not only relay the information; they also store the necessary energy to power the transmission process and provide it as needed. As essential oils interact with the lipophilic segments of the G proteins, they change the way in which the G proteins relay information to the brain. This is not without consequence.

Therapeutic Effects of Sensory Perception

In the Chinese perspective, which is not inclined to belittle fragrance, the dramatic impact of this transmission process is much easier to articulate. Classical applications of essential oils that emphasize their aroma aspect include the "fumigation of pestilent agents" and their use to open orifices and portals (to facilitate elimination), as well as for awakening consciousness and bringing about a change in worldview. Chinese medicine provides guidelines for efforts to determine fragrance effects of selected oils in the form of alignments between the five elements and flavor and fragrance qualities. (For a discussion of five element theory refer to any textbook on Chinese medicine.) Associations between odor qualities and the five elements are shown in the side panel.

Jeffrey Yuen contends that essential oils do not just cause sensory impressions, but that they also alter the way in which the sensory organs themselves operate. This can also be understood from the perspective of knowing that the sensory organs are situated in the sphere of wei qi and that there is a correlation between essential oils and wei qi (see chapter 6).

This leads to one of the most radical ideas of modern aromatherapy: by altering the way in which sensory impressions are perceived and transmitted to the brain, essential oils ultimately alter what we consider to be real. This means essential oils can change how we see the world—they can change our worldview. This can be of the highest significance for true healing.

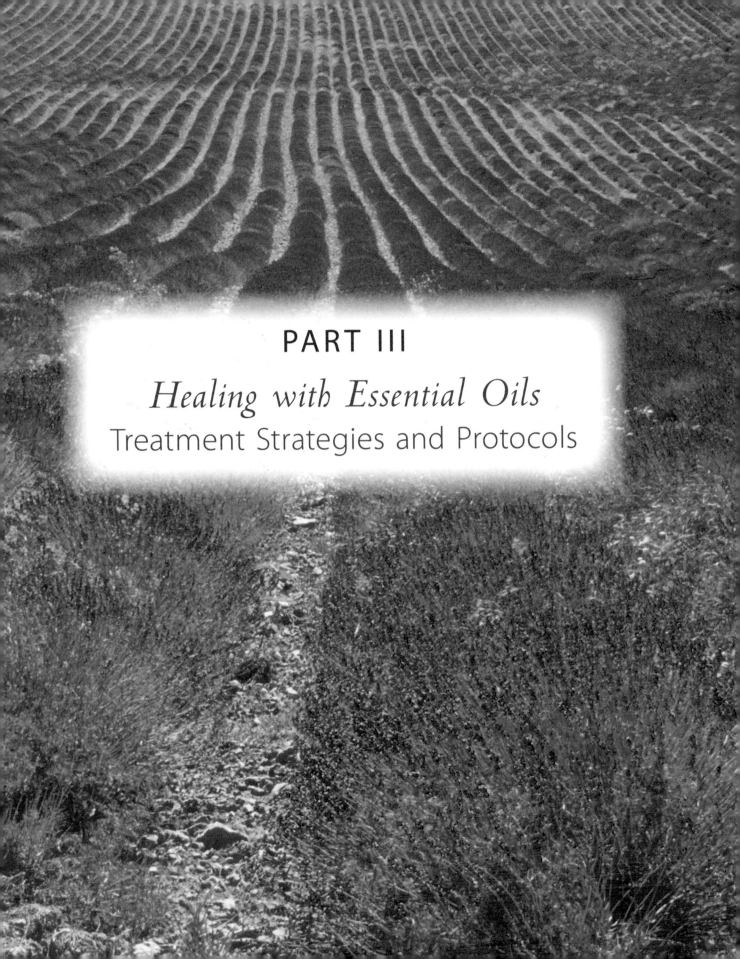

PART III

Healing with Essential Oils
Treatment Strategies and Protocols

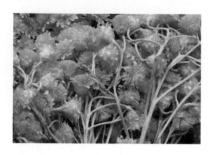

EIGHT

HOW TO APPLY ESSENTIAL OILS
Topically

The integral being cannot be a hero, or even tolerated, in a fragmented or specialist society.

MARSHALL McLUHAN AND HARLEY PARKER,
THROUGH THE VANISHING POINT

Buying an oil is easy. Often we buy an oil following an impulse. We may have read a write-up about some desirable properties or we just followed our nose to a brilliant natural fragrance. Once back home, we look up the descriptions of our new oil in the literature and a serious question arises: how are we going to actually use the oil?

At PIA we advocate a relaxed, commonsense attitude toward the actual application of essential oils, rather than making their use needlessly complicated by our conditioning from conventional medicine. Three times a day, before or after food—these are common first thoughts when we ponder essential oil application. Thus our first reflex often is to use essential oils like we would use pills.

Using essential oils in ways different than pills is warranted because the physical nature of oils is different from the often water-soluble and powdery form of most drugs. Since essential oils are mobile, lipophilic liquids, it is only logical to use them according to those qualities: common sense suggests mixing an essential oil with a fatty base oil to be used as a massage oil, therapeutic ointment, or simply a body oil for grooming. An important part of aromatherapy is learning that there is plenty of room to comfortably explore potential applications.

Some general ways in which essential oils are applied or delivered are on the skin, by ingestion or inhalation, or in the form of suppositories. Many of the most beneficial applications of an essential oil require nothing more than putting it in a base oil (see below) and applying this mixture on those areas of the body where we want its effect, such as over an organ we want to treat or on the legs for sore muscles after a bike ride. The fact that they are liquid and oily means that it is also easy to use essential oils in the shower or in the bath.

Many books describing blending and manufacture of aromatherapy preparations are available. Here we want to give a minimum of guidelines for making aromatherapy remedies at home. The recipes are kept general to serve as blueprints for many different conditions.

We are also fortunate to present selections adapted from two lectures given by naturopathic physician Dr. Pam Taylor at the 7th Scientific Aromatherapy Conference in February 2009 in San Francisco. In "Clinical Uses of Essential Oils in a Naturopathic Practice" she provided general recipes for simple essential oil applications. These are not necessarily new, but—as suggestions from a practicing naturopath—they give the aromatherapy newcomer the assurance that these recipes are in fact tried and proven. The same is true for recipes from her lecture "Essential Oils to Address Chemotherapy Side-Effects," which will be discussed in chapter 13.

Dr. Pam Taylor: Topical Preparations

While essential oils can be given orally, they are often equally effective applied topically or inhaled. This presents an advantage when the digestive system is compromised or the patient is unable to take oral dosing. This may include resistant infants or small children, individuals who find herbal remedies distasteful, or those who have difficulty swallowing.

Essential oils are rarely used undiluted. They blend best with other oils but can also be diluted in alcohol, vinegar, witch hazel, or a cream, lotion, or ointment. They may even be used with water. The liquid, cream, or ointment to which the essential oils are added is called the *carrier base* or simply *base*.

To make a preparation for use on the skin (i.e., topical), add 10 to

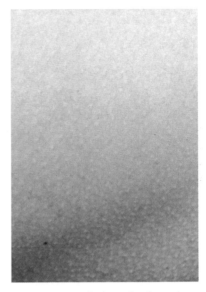

Applying essential oils on the skin is the easiest form of delivery.

CONTRIBUTORS TO AROMATHERAPY

Pam Taylor

Dr. Taylor is a practicing naturopathic physician in Moline, Illinois. She began integrating essential oils and aromatherapy into her practice many years ago. Her contribution to aromatherapy is hard to overestimate, as her extensive practical experience of using essential oils in a physician's practice is of the highest value to all the lay practitioners of aromatherapy. She has published *Simple Ways of Healing*, a textbook of natural therapies, a treasure trove for every reader interested in natural healing.[1]

How to Apply Essential Oils: Topically

Dr. Pam Taylor's Note of Caution

Anyone can react to anything, and that includes natural substances. Before using any preparation, test a small patch on the hand or foot to make sure there is no adverse reaction. Usually a reaction will manifest fairly quickly. However, be watchful for up to twenty-four hours as some reactions may be delayed.

When I prepare a blend for a patient, I always test it on my skin first, no matter how many times I've made and used the same formula before. Then I apply a small amount to the patient's hand and watch for any signs of irritation or reaction, such as redness or itching. If there is any adverse reaction to the preparation, don't use it! Because essential oils are volatile and used in small amounts, adverse reactions are generally mild and resolve quickly.

General Measure

In the recipes on the following pages, essential oil quantities are typically given per 1 ounce of base oil, unless otherwise noted. Depending on the preferred system of measurement, an ounce is approximately equal to 2 tablespoons or 30 milliliters.

20 drops of essential oil per ounce of carrier oil, cream or lotion, alcohol, witch hazel, or vinegar. Apple cider vinegar is preferable, but grain, rice, or wine vinegar will also work. For a simple and quick application, place a few drops of essential oil on a folded washcloth or small towel wrung out in cool water and apply over the affected area. Be sure to keep essential oils away from the eyes and sensitive areas of the body.

Suitable carrier oils include apricot kernel oil, sweet almond oil, safflower oil, sesame oil, Jojoba, or a light olive oil. Castor oil can be tacky and difficult to remove. However, it is anti-inflammatory and penetrates tissue well, so consider making it 5 percent of your carrier blend, that is, ¼ teaspoon (or 1.5 ml) per ounce.

Unless otherwise noted, for individuals who are frail or for babies and children under seven years of age, begin with a 1 percent dilution, that is, 7 to 10 drops of essential oil per ounce (2 tablespoons/30 ml) of carrier base. For other individuals, a 2 percent dilution of 14 to 20 drops of essential oil per ounce of carrier base may be used. Until you are familiar with the effects of the oils, start with less. You can always add more. If you find the blend is too strong, simply dilute with more carrier base.

Recipe

Sample Formula to Make a 2% Essential Oil Blend

To one fluid ounce (2 tablespoons/30 ml) carrier oil, cream, or other base, add:

    4 drops Lavender

    3 drops German (Blue) Chamomile

    2 drops Peppermint

    2 drops Ginger

    1 drop Lemon

    2 drops Cardamom

Use just enough of the blend to lightly cover the skin, moving the hands in gentle circles or in a light stroking motion. After applying essential oil blends to the skin, the bulk of the oils will be eliminated in about an hour and a half, so for persistent symptoms they may be reapplied frequently. Otherwise apply as needed.

When working with babies and small children, applying the blend to the feet, lower legs, and back reduces the risk of the oil getting into the mouth or eyes. Still, at worst getting essential oils into the mouth would be unpleasant to the taste. A dilute blend might cause some irritation to the eyes, which should clear as the essential oils evaporate.

For those who are bedridden, bandaged, clothed, or covered so that the back and tummy areas are not accessible, apply the blend to their hands, wrists, feet, and ankles. It will only take a minute or two longer for the essential oils to reach the affected areas.

Liniments

A liniment rub is refreshing, invigorating, and useful for muscle soreness or to relieve cramping in the limbs or trunk area. Add up to 10 drops of essential oil to apple cider vinegar, witch hazel hydrosol, rose water, orange water, or rubbing alcohol. Shake before each use and apply as needed to the affected area. Rubs with essential oils such as Chamomile, Ginger, Lavender, Nutmeg, and Rosemary relieve muscle spasm and pain, inducing a state of relaxation. A blend of Peppermint and Rosemary will be invigorating and help relieve depression.

Creams, Lotions, and Infused Oils

Creams, lotions, and oils are soothing and moisturizing. Add up to 10 drops of essential oil to each ounce (2 tablespoons/30 ml) of light cream or lotion. Neutral creams and lotions are readily available over the counter at health food stores or pharmacies. Find one with a basic formula whose ingredients are as natural as possible with few or no additives. Individual preference can dictate whether or not to use a lotion that is scented or unscented. Do not use products containing synthetic fragrances.

To make an infused oil, add up to 10 drops of essential oil to each ounce of a neutral carrier oil, such as apricot kernel or sweet almond oil. Olive oil, sesame oil, or safflower oils may also be used. Jojoba (a wax that is liquid at room temperature rather than an oil) has a composition similar to the sebum that coats our skin, minimal odor, and is well tolerated by those with sensitive skin. Depending on the essential oil and the tolerance of the patient, amounts ranging from 1 to 30 drops of essential oil may be added to each ounce (2 tablespoons/30 ml) of base oil.

The oil infusion is best kept in a dark glass container. If it is in

Caution

Some oils, such as Lemon and Peppermint, are quite strong, or have a potential for irritating the mucous membranes or skin in higher concentrations. It is best to use only 1 or 2 drops of these oils per ounce of carrier base, even if no other essential oils are added.

How to Apply Essential Oils:
Topically

Absorption

For a while the question of whether or not and to what extent essential oils are absorbed into the body via the skin was hotly contested. This often-irrational debate shall not be revisited here. The fact is that ultimately experimental science was able to establish that essential oil components applied to the skin of a test person did show up in the bloodstream of that person, even after the nose was clipped shut with a clothespin and breathing air was funneled in from an oil-free space.

The more interesting question, of whether and how effectively all or almost all components of an essential oil are absorbed, has not been answered by experimental science. The requisite setup, one that can check for hundreds of components simultaneously, has not yet been realized.

For the purposes of common sense it is sufficient to recognize that essential oil components are absorbed into the body via the skin, some faster and some slower, and some maybe not at all.

clear glass, keep the infusion in a cool, dark place to lengthen its shelf life. The oil should be usable and potent for several months. Check the oil periodically for any rancid odor or cloudiness, indicating spoilage or microbial contamination. If this occurs do not use the oil. Throw it away.

Essential Oils in the Bath

Create a soothing and therapeutic bath by adding 2 cups (550 ml) of Epsom salt and 8 to 10 drops of essential oils to the bath water. Epsom salt contains magnesium, a natural antidepressant and muscle relaxant, whose benefits are best realized with a soak of 20 minutes or longer. The sulfate molecule helps power detoxification pathways in the liver. If the patient's skin is dry, omit the Epsom salt or rinse off the bath water with the shower head.

After getting out of the bath, pat the skin dry with a towel to remove excess water, leaving the skin moist. Apply a light fatty oil or moisturizer to help the skin retain the water absorbed during bathing. Do not add bath oil to the bath water, as this will coat the skin and inhibit the absorption of the Epsom salt and essential oils. Epsom salt is useful in correcting heart arrhythmias, is a bronchodilator, helps reduce the frequency and severity of asthma attacks, relieves pain associated with fibromyalgia, arthritis, and muscle soreness, and can modify the severity of symptoms associated with shingles.

If the individual is unable to use a bathtub, a sheet wrap may be prepared by adding 2 cups of Epsom salt to 2 gallons of warm or comfortably hot water along with the desired essential oils. After laying down plastic to protect the bedding, wring out the sheet, and wrap the individual from the shoulders to the feet. Cover the person with a wool or Vellux blanket, placing a bolster or rolled towel under the knees to reduce back strain. Allow him or her to rest for 20 minutes, or until a mild sweat is produced. Remove the wrap and use a cool water sponge bath to remove the sweat and Epsom salt. Pat the skin dry and cover the person with a fresh sheet and blanket, and allow him or her to rest for at least 20 minutes.

Using Essential Oils in the Shower

An effective, pleasant, and truly effortless way to use oils is to apply them to the skin during a shower. This form of application allows the use of larger quantities of oil, somewhere between 5 and 20 drops per application. Start with less if you are not sure how a specific oil will be tolerated. Once we have clearly established that the reactions caused by a specific essential oil are pleasant, we can go ahead and use it more liberally in the shower.

This application is particularly easy. In many cases essential oils can be used straight out of the bottle. These casual uses of essential oils may in fact be the most beneficial to every essential oil user's health, because they employ the many simultaneous effects of secondary metabolites to maintain balanced immuno-vigilance and prevent many conditions from developing in the first place. Many common essential oils can be used out of the bottle in the shower or dabbed on the skin.

We suggest using those oils that can be applied undiluted, rather than mixed in with a base oil. The application of the straight essential oil on the wet skin without a fatty oil component will have a particular glistening and effective character. The essential oil will be absorbed into the skin tissue immediately. With many oils a characteristic and pleasant tingle will occur and no reminiscent oil film will remain after rinsing and toweling off.

To apply an oil in the shower, turn off the water halfway through and distribute a few drops on the wet skin. Clearly, the oil will not mix with the water on the skin. This is, however, not a problem but an advantage. As the oil is repulsed by the water, its tendency to be absorbed into the lipophilic (fatty) skin tissue will increase. Still, the water will help make it easy to work the oil over the whole body (if that is desired), so that every square inch of skin can be used as an absorbing surface.

If you have never done this before, start by putting only 2 drops behind the knee and then work the oil upward on your wet skin. Only when you know positively that an oil is tolerated well, and you have incrementally increased the amount of oil you are using, should the full amount of oil as indicated in the following description be used. Begin with the feet: top and soles receive a drop each. Continue upward on the shin and calf by putting a drop on the outside shin just below the

CONTRIBUTORS TO AROMATHERAPY

Monika Haas

Monika Haas has developed what can be termed "preventive aromatherapy." Because of the many physiological effects of essential oils—such as their capacity to induce detoxification, their ability to moderate inflammation, or their role in maintaining balance within the autonomic nervous system—their use in daily life provides a degree of prevention that is hard to overestimate. She has greatly expanded the scope of aromatherapy by developing formulations that offer exquisite preventive efficacy along with highly pleasant forms of application during normal daily activities. Two examples illustrate the approach: taking a shower is seized as an opportunity for the refreshing use of an immune-boosting formula and brushing one's teeth is completed with a mouthwash, maintaining oral hygiene.

How to Apply Essential Oils: Topically

Testing for Irritation

The essential oils listed in the "Essential Oils for the Shower" section are generally most gentle. In some cases they cause a tingle, but one that is sufficiently gentle so they can still be used casually in the shower.

Nonetheless, anyone can react to anything. It is absolutely essential to test and retest whenever a new oil or a new batch is tried. A drop or two are applied to the hand or inside of the elbow and watched for signs of irritation. Only when we know an oil creates a desirable sensation is it safe to slightly increase the number of drops used per shower.

knee, then a drop each over the lymph nodes, left and right, in the groin area. Then another drop or two are put on the solar plexus, over the liver, and 2 to 5 drops distributed over the chest and abdominal area. Apply 1 to 2 drops over the lymph nodes in the underarm area and possibly another drop or two on the throat area. If you like the sensation of the oil, you can also make a quick swish over the face, not applying another drop but simply distributing what is already on the hands from before.

Oils used in this way need to be gentle and pleasant enough to give this procedure more of a playful rather than a medicinal character (see below for a list of oils appropriate to use in the shower). This form of application serves to connect with the plant world in the morning before we start our day. It is also a easy way to explore the different layers of quality of an essential oil (see "Lavender Authenticity" in chapter 5, pages 86–91).

For the novice it is a good idea to try the application of essential oils in the shower with Lavender oil first. Because of its extremely mild nature, Lavender works well for becoming familiarized with this form of liberal oil use without the risk of irritation. As we become familiar with different essential oils and with this form of application, we develop a good sense of which oils to try in this fashion.

Essential Oils for the Shower

The recommendations for oils suited for the shower pertain to truly authentic essential oils. They should be refreshing and gentle for easy use directly on the skin.

> **Bay Laurel:** lymph and general tonic; may cause sensitivity if overused (longer than 7 days)
>
> **Black Spruce:** adrenal tonic; especially effective if distributed over the lower back
>
> **Cape Chamomile:** de-stressing; crisp fragrance and soothing, nonirritant, nature make it particularly carefree
>
> **Cardamom:** prevents cramping; completely nonirritant
>
> **Clary Sage:** relaxing and nurturing; nonirritant
>
> **Coriander Seed:** tonic; the best Coriander Seed oils are complex and fragrant

Cypress: decongestant

Douglas Fir: tonic; some batches of needle oils may be irritant

Eucalyptus radiata: Mild on the skin; strong antiviral effect

Geranium: nurturing; there are many different qualities on the market, and some may be slightly more tingling than others

Hyssop decumbens: nerve tonic, prevents infection, and eases breathing; nonirritant

Lavandin: balancing and cleansing; may be slightly stimulating for some individuals; different qualities on the market may cause different degrees of tingle

Lavender: relaxing and cleansing

Monarda: radiant tonic and powerful emotional uplift; comes with some tingle, which may be too strong for some skin types, so it can be diluted with some Lavandin

Myrtle: tonifies lungs and thyroid; most gentle on the skin

Niaouli (*Melaleuca quinquenervi viridiflora* **or MQV**): invigorating; the extremely broad—multitarget and multicomponent—activity of this essential oil is best explored in the shower application

Palmarosa: immunoboosting; this oil has a somewhat viscous consistency and may be too strong for some

Petitgrain: de-stressing; of the many qualities on the market, the best are totally nonirritant

Pine: common adrenal tonic; authentic oils are nonirritant, but different provenances can be found on the market and need to be tested for irritation

Ravintsara: immunoboost, nerve tonic; totally nonirritant

Rose: nerve tonic; may have a tingle or slight scratch on certain skin types

Rosemary verbenone: mucolytic; nonirritant

Sage petit feuilles: strengthening; nonirritant

Spike Lavender: immunoboost, heart tonic; authentic oils are nonirritant

Tea Tree: cleansing; should be nonirritant, but check for irritation

Thyme linalool: candida prevention; may have a pleasant tingle

Thyme thuyanol: cleansing immunoboost; can develop some warmth on certain skin types, but is ultimately well tolerated

Casual Selection of Oils

It is exactly their simplicity that makes casual essential oil application styles so useful for daily prevention and immunomaintenance. Because they are so simple and require almost no time, most aromatherapy enthusiasts will in fact utilize them and thereby really derive the benefits. It is not necessary to have a precise indication in order to use an oil in the shower. You can look at the range of essential oils available at the moment and then choose the one that feels most attractive.

Characteristics of Some Oils when Used in the Shower

Following are some examples of what can be expected when oils are used in the shower.

Palmarosa, the Antiviral Agent

Palmarosa creates a strong tingling sensation, which leaves a thorough impression on mind and body. This oil, although intrinsically mild, may be too strong for some and should be mixed with a very soft oil such as Lavender.

Niaouli Provides Good Immune Support

Niaouli oil helps to avoid catching a cold when the other members of the household are already sneezing or are sick with flu. Used in the shower, the oil develops an interesting spectrum of fragrance going from an initial pungent monoterpene impact to an interesting study of not-so-familiar sesquiterpene notes. This oil presents the open-minded individual with an interesting learning opportunity. The unfamiliar notes in this oil become more and more likeable as we become aware of its benefits. It thus stimulates essential oil intuition.

Bay Laurel Moves the Lymph

The topical application of Bay Laurel is an effective way to keep the lymph moving. The sensation that Bay Laurel leaves after a shower is hard to describe. It is just the right measure of gentle stimulation to teach a commonsense attitude toward secondary plant metabolites: easy does it. For instance, there may be times when you crave a daily shower with Bay Laurel. While it is fine to give in to that urge for a while, there will also be a moment when you forget to use the oil. It is important not to react with self-punishment or to try and somehow make up for the missed application. Forgetting an oil is generally a sign that our body is content.

Such an on/off approach apparently suits the immune system much better than continuously going through the same routine with a puritan sense of duty. In the case of Bay Laurel, excessive use—day in and day out for more than a week or two—can actually lead to a certain sensitivity to the oil, and what was once tolerated without problem can suddenly start to cause slight itches.

Dabbing and Rubbing: Undiluted Topical Applications

As with the application of undiluted essential oils in the shower, essential oils need to be tested for irritation before dabbing or rubbing them on. The gradual exploration of the actual interaction of our own skin type and condition with essential oils will create the confidence to use them when we really need to! A significant benefit from using undiluted essential oils, which escapes scientific experiments, is the visceral and physiological experience we accumulate whenever we use essential oils in this fashion. Of course, only authentic essential oils can be used undiluted without annoying irritation.

As we test different essential oils on the skin we develop different layers of experience. We build a fairly reliable sphere of intuition that guides us and tells us that Lavender and Ravintsara are easy to use on the skin. Equally well we know that Mountain Savory will further inflame any red spots we have and we will learn to be extra careful when checking out new provenances of needle or citrus oils. Last but not least we will build a fairly good understanding of the relative quality of different commercial sources, as some suppliers generally deal in authentic essential oils and others in standardized fare. The difference will be obvious once these oils are put on the skin.

Dabbing

Dabbing is best explained with the treatment suggestion for facial herpes. To treat herpes, the oil or oil blend is applied directly onto the lesions. This can be done with a Q-tip or simply by dabbing a drop onto the lesion with the finger. This is repeated frequently at the beginning of the treatment. (Doing this 5 to 10 times on the first day of treatment is fine.) Fever blisters inside the mouth can be treated in exactly the same way. In this case it is advantageous to use *Hyssop decumbens,* as its taste and feel inside the mouth is somewhat more agreeable than the turpentine explosions set off by many other essential oils. Even though there is no adverse effect attached to these turpentine explosions, they require a certain amount of getting used to until they are tolerated or even appreciated with a shrug.

Massive Rub

Since the influenza virus replicates in the tissues of the nose and throat, but also deep within the lung tissue, French-style aromatherapy suggests the topical application of substantial amounts of essential oil. The intent is to keep the concentration of essential oils as high as possible in the body, especially the bloodstream. This is meant to inactivate the virus as it travels from one cell to another. Whether this strategy really succeeds is unclear. It is not really known whether the essential oil concentrations in the bloodstream are high enough to inactivate (destroy) viruses as they shuttle from an already destroyed cell to a fresh one.

The classic practice is to apply essential oils by rubbing them on the torso, up to 2 ml (or approximately 40 to 50 drops) per session, up to five sessions per day. Essential oils especially suited for rubs to treat the flu are *Eucalyptus radiata, Eucalyptus dives,* Spike Lavender, and Thyme thuyanol. The effectiveness of these treatments is increased by frequent inhalations and, if fever and severity of the condition necessitate, delivering essential oils via suppositories.

Essential Oils Used Undiluted Locally

Mild undiluted essential oils can be appropriate in the treatment of localized skin issues and to deliver larger quantities of essential oil for systemic issues.

Angelica Root: 3 drops on the solar plexus will help prepare for sleep; this essential oil can be photosensitizing, so do not use topically in the sun

Bay Laurel: a few drops can be spread over the lymph nodes

German Chamomile: dab on inflamed spots for quick action; using the oil diluted is equally effective

Roman Chamomile: apply to solar plexus, neck, and shoulder muscles

Everlasting: very effective in diluted form, but the oil can be used undiluted for quick action to treat emergencies, cuts, sports or other injuries; open wounds should be treated with pure Helichrysum essential oil to avoid complications from getting fatty oil into an open sore

Inula graveolens: a drop or two, diluted or undiluted, applied over the heart area should relieve constriction and ease breathing

Lavender: use for mosquito bites, or apply a few drops to the neck for relaxation

Katrafay: muscle pain

Khella: a single drop applied to solar plexus and sternum area will ease constriction; it is equally or more effective when diluted

Neroli: 1 drop dabbed anywhere, such as the sternum area, will ease anxiety

Peppermint: dabbed on dull injuries, ideally combined with ice, will prevent swelling

Rose: can be dabbed on temples or wrists, as perfume or as a fragrant tonic

Thuja: can be dabbed on warts; care should be used to avoid healthy skin as much as possible

Thyme thuyanol: anywhere

Vitex: a single drop applied to wrists or temples will provide the hormonal rebalancing effect of this plant

Ylang-Ylang: a drop or two dispersed over the heart area will relax and calm

Caution with Higher Dosages

Higher dosages of essential oil should only be utilized after you have gradually built the necessary experience with such doses, enabling you to know which essential oils you can tolerate in this fashion.

The Power of Dilution: Applications with a Base Oil

It is important to realize that the main reason to use nonirritant essential oils undiluted is generally convenience. The assumption that undiluted essential oils will work more efficiently is generally not true. Perhaps surprisingly, experience often indicates that diluted oil is more effective than undiluted. Such observations can be explained chemically in that certain molecules rearrange into less active forms when they are present in high concentration. The molecule curls up because it sees too many of its own kind. Diluted, it sees more molecules from other oils and it relaxes into a more stretched out and active form. It appears that

How to Apply Essential Oils: Topically

increased efficacy upon dilution is a phenomenon observed mostly with authentic oils.

As convenient as it may be to take a drop of essential oil directly out of the bottle, there are situations where dilution with a base oil (such as sesame, hazelnut, or almond oil) is preferred (see "Sample Formula to Make a 2% Essential Oil Blend" on page 120). For actual treatments it is often necessary to apply essential oils over long periods of time. Intuition suggests that in such cases a stock bottle with essential oils diluted in a base oil should be prepared.

Other Diluting Agents

A condition where dilution is key is eczema. However, fatty oils are often not the choice of eczema patients, as their oily feel is perceived as distressing. For eczema treatments it is best to integrate essential oils into a non-oily base. One possibility is to use a water-based acrylic gel; even though such gels are synthetic, they provide an effective and convenient means of delivery. Dogmatic insistence on natural carrier materials often leads to abandoning the treatment and may be self-defeating.

An easy way to prepare essential oil remedies for eczema treatments without the potentially cumbersome procurement of acrylic gels is to mix the essential oil component with Aloe Vera gel. Another option is to disperse a drop of the undiluted blend with the help of some hydrosols such as Myrtle, Lavender, or Everlasting.

NINE

HOW TO APPLY ESSENTIAL OILS
Internally

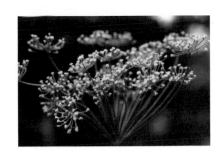

The skill of nations depends on their food.

BRILLAT-SAVARIN

Comparing Topical and Internal Use

Ingesting essential oils is a topic at the center of one of aromatherapy's culture wars. Let us again try to diffuse some of the tension with common sense. Despite conventional assumptions, topical application of essential oils can be highly effective, as they penetrate lipophilic (fatty) skin tissue effectively and even enter the bloodstream via this route. They will be metabolized eventually once they reach the liver.

Ingested essential oils, on the other hand, reach the liver very quickly where they are metabolized and eliminated. It is advantageous to ingest an essential oil only if the metabolic intermediates produced during elimination create a desired therapeutic effect and safety parameters are favorable.

Ingesting: The Easy Way

The discussion about the safety and overall usefulness of ingesting essential oils has gone on for a long time; it consists mainly of a superficial back and forth of talking points provided by different parties with vested interests. Obviously those engaged in the manufacture

131

Essential Oils Are Not Pills

It is instructive to repeat the very obvious: essential oils are liquid, oily (fat soluble), volatile, and fragrant. The best modes of application derive from the recognition of these physical qualities.

and distribution of adulterated oils, knowing about the added natural or synthetic chemicals, will warn against ingesting essential oils. It appears, however, that ingesting a drop of such oils is harmless, based on all the experience gathered in aromatherapy and from what is known about the toxicity of quite a number of essential oils.

Common sense helps to resolve the issue. While there are essential oils that are toxic when ingested (see chapter 5, "Aromatherapy Safety in the Information Age"), the question immediately arises: should, for example, authentic Lemon oil not be ingested just because adulterated essential oils may contain harmful chemicals, or because some ketone-containing essential oils may be toxic? In other words, limiting the discussion to a general "ingestion yes" or an "ingestion no" misses the point.

The questions that need to be answered are which essential oils can be ingested and what is the benefit? On the facing page you will find a list of essential oils suitable for casual ingestion in a glass of water, and the benefits that can be derived from them. As stated previously, one benefit lies in building a repertoire of personal physiological experience with essential oils. These experiences will be most valuable when circumstances indeed call for ingesting an oil. Because we have already built up a body of physiological recognition, we no longer wrestle with the concept of ingesting essential oils.

How to Ingest

For those who do ingest essential oils, the actual mechanics or technique of ingestion is very much an individual matter. Many people prefer to simply slurp or lick the essential oil off a teaspoon. This is, however, only of limited efficacy. A drop of essential oil ingested in this manner will be absorbed mostly into the mucous membranes of the mouth and throat and maybe the esophagus, potentially delaying its absorption into the liver.

A most effective method is to put a drop of oil in a glass of water. Quite a number of oils will form a very fine film on top of the water. Vigorous stirring will not really dissolve the drop but will disperse it sufficiently so that drinking the glass of water will take the oil into the stomach and ideally into the small intestine. Another method is to disperse a drop of oil in a teaspoon of honey. The honey can then be dissolved in water or eaten as is; this will also transport the oil to the small intestine.

The French aromatherapy literature contains many references to using oils orally. The suggested procedure is to put the essential oils into a gel capsule that is stomach acid resistant. Use of a gel cap typically requires that the essential oil first be dissolved in a carrier oil and then the capsule is filled with the appropriate amount of the mixture. Clearly many casual users will be discouraged by this suggestion.

Essential Oils Suited for Casual Ingestion in a Glass of Water

Dosage: Generally 1 drop is always enough when ingesting essential oils. However, sometimes inadvertently more than 1 drop of essential oil will come out of the bottle. Such slightly higher doses are normally well tolerated and there is no need to prepare a fresh glass.

Anise Seed: 1 to 3 drops on a sugar cube or in a glass of water stabilize heartbeat and breathing

Bay Laurel: 1 drop; stimulant, anti-infectious

Cardamom: 1 drop will help digestion but also ease emotional upset

Carrot Seed: 1 to 3 drops can be taken sporadically or as part of a program of liver regeneration

Celery Seed: can be taken once or twice, 3 days in a row, to drain toxicity from the kidneys

German Chamomile: can be taken in almost any amount to calm the stomach and helps with COPD (chronic obstructive pulmonary disease)

Cinnamon Bark: 1 drop on a sugar cube, once every 2 hours, for acute tropical infections

Coriander Seed: carminative and tonic

Cypress: nervous cough

Dill: childhood colic, indigestion

Helichrysum: 1 drop will restart liver activity after "crise de fois" (crisis of the liver)

Fennel: 1 to 3 drops; analgesic, sedates reflexes

Frankincense: immuno deficiency and depression

Greenland Moss: 1 to 3 drops for liver regeneration

Hops: 1 drop is a powerful sedative

Ginger: digestive tonic

Goldenrod: 1 to 3 drops for nervousness, ANS imbalance

Juniper: 1 to 3 drops for pain relief, neuralgia

Lavender: eases the cravings accompanying low blood sugar

Lemon: 1 to 3 drops; induces detoxification, cleansing

Marjoram: 1 drop; slightly tranquilizing

Mastick: 1 drop; lymph and prostate decongestant

Melissa: 1 to 3 drops; deepens sleep

Myrrh: pain and inflammation, relief for gums

Oregano: 1 drop for acute tonsillitis; careful—this oil burns and needs to be absorbed on a charcoal pill or something similar that will release it slowly

Peppermint: 1 to 3 drops; nausea; absolutely not suited for children under 5

Ravintsara: 1 to 3 drops; nerve tonic, depression

Rock Rose: 1 to 3 drops; internal bleeding

Rosemary verbenone: digestive

Sage petit feuilles: regenerating, nurturing

St. John's Wort: 1 to 3 drops; slightly euphoric

Tarragon: 1 to 3 drops; shock

Tea Tree: 1 to 3 drops; cystitis

Thyme thuyanol: 1 to 3 drops; anti-infectious, stimulant, but not overly so

Vitex: PMS, menopause

Tea Tree Oil for Cystitis

A condition that responds quickly to the uncomplicated "1 to 3 drops of essential oil in a glass of water" application is cystitis. Tea Tree oil can be used either by itself or in a premade blend of 20 parts Tea Tree oil with 1 part Mountain Savory. One to 3 drops of the essential oil or the blend are drunk repeatedly during the day. In the beginning of an acute condition, this can be done every 20 minutes and the symptoms will diminish quickly. Then the frequency of consumption of the Tea Tree drink can be reduced. Treating cystitis with Tea Tree oil is highly effective. Nonetheless, if the cystitis is recurrent, diet or lifestyle changes may be required for a full resolution.

Ingesting Lemon Oil and Liver Detoxification

A Drop of Oil in a Glass of Water

Lemon essential oil is nontoxic, provided it is organic and free of pesticides. Its taste is relatively mild and noninvasive. These two factors make Lemon oil the perfect choice for everyone who wants to explore ingesting essential oils. However, it is very important to use only organic Lemon oil, as all Citrus oils are cold pressed, and if there are pesticides on the peel they will directly flow into the essential oil.

The experiment is simple: 1 to 3 drops of Lemon oil are added to a glass of water and stirred. It does not matter whether the oil is still dispersed while drinking the water or if the oil has partially accumulated again at the surface. Some of the oil will most likely remain in the water glass. In any case, sufficient quantities of essential oil will reach the stomach and ultimately the liver, producing its balanced inhibition and the induction of liver detoxification enzymes.

The objective of this little experiment is to begin learning the range of sensations and physiological responses we receive from ingesting essential oils. Over time this will create awareness of the effects essential oils can have on physiological systems such as the ANS, the digestive tract, or the lymphatic system.

Caution First-Time Users

Ingesting Lemon oil is known as an entirely harmless exercise to many aromatherapy users. Nonetheless, it is imperative that the first time user explore this application simply with 1 drop. Essential oils are very powerful, concentrated messengers from the plant world. For those not used to the detoxification effect, the oil may trigger slight anxiety due to unfamiliar sensations. It is important to proceed cautiously in the quest for experience.

Essential Oils and Phase I Liver Detoxification

Many xenobiotics are oily and not soluble in water and tend to accumulate in body tissues, especially adipose tissue. As we have seen, evolution has generated a mechanism by which these substances can be removed from the organism. For anyone interested in optimum health, this mechanism can be employed to prevent the accumulation of toxic levels of these xenobiotics. It is done simply by ingesting an essential oil such as Lemon oil, which will trigger or modify the detoxification process.

The process starts with Phase I, in which the essential molecules or toxins are made water soluble and more responsive to further elimination reactions by Phase II enzymes.

The Phase I or CYP 450 enzyme systems can catalyze almost any reaction a compound can undergo. CYP 450 enzymes are located in liver smooth endoplasmic reticulum, the gut mucosa, and also in smaller amounts in airway mucosa, and in the kidneys, skin, and brain. These enzyme systems are directed primarily at endogenous compounds and dietary xenobiotics. The fact that they also metabolize drugs is a consequence of their broad (nonselective) reactivity.

Inhalation

Inhalation does not have to be complicated. As a matter of fact, the easier one keeps the procedure the more likely it will have benefits. Given the volatile nature of essential oils, putting them in the air is easy. Putting a drop of essential oil on a piece of paper towel and inhaling it is effective. Putting a drop of essential oil on a pillow overnight is highly effective and requires practically no effort. Besides directly inhaling them, essential oils can also be used more ambiantly. Diffusing them into rooms will lower the count of airborne microorganisms significantly, reducing the risk of infection especially in offices and waiting rooms. Diffusing essential oils in rooms and houses has even been reported to be effective in expelling mold from infested buildings.

According to Dr. Pam Taylor, when oils are inhaled they interact with cells at the back of the nose to stimulate a change in the areas of the brain that control nausea and vomiting as well as sleep and mood.

Essential Oil Suppositories

Suppositories are a prickly topic in many cultural environments. It is typically mothers, with their practicality, who start concocting suppositories when the seriousness of a child's condition and lack of better options create enough of an incentive. Applying essential oils by means of suppository often has stunning therapeutic benefits. One main advantage of essential oil suppositories is their capacity to safely deliver essential oils that would otherwise be too irritant. The suggestion of essential oil suppositories originates from French-style aromatherapy, which has found them to be hugely effective in the treatment of serious acute and chronic bronchitis. The French literature on medical aromatherapy is full of suggestions for suppository formulas for a wide variety of conditions. *L'aromathérapie exactement* lists a fair number of essential oil synergies specifically for suppositories and the treatment of a variety of symptoms.[1]

As the essential oils delivered by suppository make their way first and foremost to the lungs, French-style aromatherapy also employs suppositories to prevent or counter asthma attacks. Experience shows that the typical antiasthmatic essential oils will ease an attack, but in the case of an adult, not really break it up. Since there are some potential complications

Essential Oil Inhalation

Using essential oils as inhalants provides an effective application that can continue while an individual rests or sleeps.

Diffusers distribute the oils by dispersing them into the air as a very fine mist.

If a diffuser is not available, place 3 to 5 drops of a single oil or blend of oils on a cotton ball and place the cotton ball near the bed, or place several treated cotton balls throughout the living space. The treated cotton ball can also be carried in a small plastic bag to open and use as needed, for example when riding in a car or on a plane.

Alternatively, place a small amount of salt, sand, or Epsom salt in a bowl or small jar that has a wide mouth and add 10 or 15 drops of a single essential oil or a blend of oils. The salt will slow down the evaporation of the oils, making them effective over a longer period of time. A spice jar works well for this method; use the ones that come with a plastic "sifter" top that has holes in it in addition to the lid. The sifter top reduces spillage if the bottle is knocked over.

when using essential oils on asthma patients who have no prior experience with essential oils, this topic is left to more specialized study.

Why Suppositories?

Deep-seated and severe chronic bronchitis reacts quickly to treatment with essential oils when delivered by suppositories. The uninitiated will ask, why suppositories? The answer is that this method delivers the essential oils directly to the lung tissues where they are, in cases of stubborn bronchitis, needed the most: the lower bronchial capillaries. Essential oils absorbed into the abdominal veins bypass the liver. They are fed directly into the heart-lung circulatory system without first being subjected to biotransformation by the liver detoxification enzyme system. Consequently, they reach the lower bronchial capillaries in their original lipophilic and volatile state, still capable of eliminating pathogenic microorganisms and dissolving and expectorating mucus.

Ingested essential oils are absorbed into the liver before they can reach the lungs. In this case the oils are metabolized by liver detoxification enzymes into a water-soluble form. Once essential oils are converted into water-soluble compounds their antimicrobial, mucolytic, and expectorant qualities may be lost or reduced.

Essential Oils for Suppositories

Suppositories are perfectly suited to treat small children and babies. The rectal application of essential oils in suppositories avoids the strong sensations of fragrance and taste associated with other forms of delivery. It should be understood that only essential oils that are 100 percent authentic, nontoxic, and nonirritant should be considered. To treat acute and chronic bronchitis and cough in infants the essential oil of *Hyssop decumbens* (CAUTION: It is absolutely critical not to confuse this oil with the toxic *Hyssop officinalis*) or *Thymus vulgaris* of the geraniol type have proven to be very successful (CAUTION: Do not confuse with the irritant phenol types of Thyme).

For adults the spectrum of essential oils that can be used in suppositories is much broader (see page 138). Typically, adults resort to suppositories only when confronted with stubborn or seriously acute bronchitis, often accompanied by fever. These conditions frequently have a strong bacterial component. The suppository route is

The Suppository Trick: Veins Deliver Essential Oils Directly to the Lungs

The heart pulls oxygen-depleted blood from the veins into the heart-lung circulatory system. When essential oils have been absorbed into the abdominal veins they travel with the oxygen-depleted blood. They reach the heart, which pumps the depleted blood to the lungs, where it is recharged with oxygen. This is the route by which suppository-delivered essential oils reach the lung tissue so quickly and directly! Oxygen-rich blood is pulled back from the lungs into the heart and it is then sent into the body's circulatory system.

How to Apply Essential Oils: Internally

best suited to deliver essential oils that are the strongest antibacterial agents, but difficult to apply because of their irritant character. The antibacterial essential oils of Mountain Savory, Oregano, or Cinnamon Leaf are appropriately delivered in suppositories.

Strong Anti-infectious Essential Oils Recommended in French Aromatherapy for Suppository Use

For Adults

Mountain Savory

Thymus vulgaris thymol

Oreganum compactum

These oils can be integrated into a blend for use in suppositories. Their concentration should be 2 to 3 drops per suppository, which translates into 20 to 30 drops to make 10 suppositories. The remaining 30 to 40 drops to reach the total number of drops of 60 (the suggested amount for adults) should be *Thymus vulgaris* thuyanol, *Hyssop decumbens,* Rosemary verbenone, Myrtle, or another mild oil of choice.

Another option for the forceful element of an anti-infectious suppository blend is to integrate Cinnamon Leaf and Cinnamon Bark. The suggested concentration is at the equivalent of 1 drop each per suppository; the remainder of the blend should consist of mild essential oils.

Rosemary verbenone is frequently suggested as part of a suppository blend for respiratory infections (sinusitis, rhinitis, bronchitis, etc.) for its mucolytic qualities. Because of its mild nature, it can make up as much as 50 percent of the suppository blend.

For Children

The treatment of persistent bronchitis conditions for small children (one year and older) with suppositories with the mildest anti-infectious essential oils has been very successful. Ten drops only are used to make 10 suppositories. Oils recommended by the French aromatherapy literature for small children:

Hyssop decumbens

Thymus vulgaris geraniol

Suppositories Made Easy

The need to use suppositories generally arises unforeseen in the form of a seriously acute condition. Hence it is helpful to know how they can be made without a lot of prep work. The crucial ingredient is cocoa butter. When purchasing cocoa butter it is important to find a product that in fact is only cocoa butter and does not have mineral oil, petrolatum, or paraffin added.

The standard recipe for homemade suppositories is intended to yield approximately ten suppositories. This requires 20 grams (two-thirds of an ounce) of cocoa butter and 10 ml (one-third of an ounce) of a base oil, ideally sesame oil. The measuring of these quantities can be done rather roughly. The idea is to create a mass that can be melted into a homogeneous liquid state into which the essential oils can be dissolved. Once the essential oils are dissolved the mass should easily return to the solid state once put in the freezer.

The 20-gram quantity of cocoa butter often can be eyeballed as a fraction of the original container size in which the cocoa butter was sold. Cocoa butter is often retailed in 50-gram containers; half of the contents would therefore be approximately 25 grams, which would be close enough. Ten ml of base oil can be measured, or approximated, by filling an empty 15 ml essential oil bottle approximately two-thirds full; again the rough approximation will do.

Dr. Pam Taylor on Suppositories

Essential oil suppositories can be helpful in a number of ways.

- Suppositories with essential oils such as German Chamomile, Helichrysum, and Lavender can be used to soothe inflamed or irritated vaginal or rectal tissues.
- Thyme and Oregano are highly antimicrobial.
- Ginger and Peppermint are antispasmodic and will also relieve nausea.

Watch for signs of discomfort or irritation. If irritation does occur, an enema or douche of warm water can be used to flush out the remaining essential oils and cocoa butter.

Since essential oils are eliminated out of the body tissues in 1 to 2 hours, a fresh suppository may be inserted every 1 to 2 hours if found helpful.

Recipe

Making Suppositories

Combine the cocoa butter and the sesame oil in a stainless steel kitchen pot and heat ever so gently until the cocoa butter is molten and forms a homogeneous liquid with the sesame oil. (To be most prudent it is advisable to use a double burner, that is, place the pot with the cocoa butter and the sesame oil in another, bigger pot with an inch of water in it, rather than directly on the burner. This way the water in the bigger pot is heated and the cocoa butter and sesame oil in the smaller pot are only indirectly heated via the water of the larger pot!)

Once the mass is fully liquid, add 60 drops of the desired essential oil mix for adults (10 to 20 drops for children, depending on age). It is practical to add 1 drop of German Chamomile to the essential oil blend. By its blue color it is easier to see when the oil blend is homogeneously dissolved. The mixture is then allowed to cool.

How to Apply Essential Oils: Internally

When the mixture has become waxy, but not yet brittle, scoop out ten roughly equal pieces with a teaspoon and roll them up one by one in pieces of aluminum foil (approximately 2" x 2").

Place the rolls in the freezer where they will turn solid. Remove them from the freezer and peel them out of the aluminum foil directly before their intended use.

TEN

ESSENTIAL OILS FOR COMMON AILMENTS

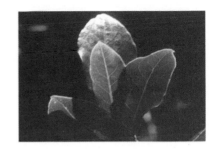

A wiser insight may be to observe that we receive the medical treatments that match our beliefs.

PAUL PITCHFORD, *HEALING WITH WHOLE FOODS*

This chapter and those that follow offer guidelines and strategies for the use of essential oils for treating diverse conditions, drawing on the different influences that have shaped the current state of aromatherapy.

Treating Infections

As essential oils target a broad variety of structural elements of functional proteins and phospholipid membranes, they are effective against viral as well as fungal or bacterial infections.

Viral Infections

Herpes

An overwhelming number of individuals find essential oils to be the best method of managing their herpes condition, often improving the immune response to the point that there are no recurrences. But not everyone has acute herpes and gathers experiences by autoexperimentation. Nonetheless, it is generally sound to pass on effective oils such as Tea Tree, Geranium, or *Eucalyptus radiata* to individuals who might appreciate a natural treatment.

It is also instructive to listen to the reports of others in the aromatherapy community. The experience accumulated over time speaks

UNDERSTANDING AROMATHERAPY

For Further Exploration

Advanced Aromatherapy is a classic text that details many of the most common treatment applications of essential oils along the lines of French-style aromatherapy.

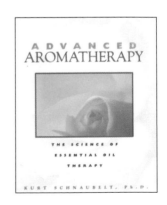

Herpes Treatment

The accepted logic that a specific drug is needed for a specific pathogen is suspended when we realize that practically all essential oils are effective against herpes lesions. There is an intuitive grasp that maybe it is the purpose of essential oils in the plant to protect against viral infection!

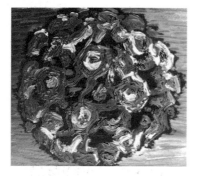

Artist's rendition of a herpes virus (original painting by Monika Haas)

a clear language. Evaluating the cumulative record, we notice that it is extremely rare that an individual will react negatively to essential oil treatment of herpes. In the rare cases that it does happen, it is most likely for reasons of having a particularly disturbed immune response.

Shingles

The treatment of shingles (herpes zoster) with essential oils is equally successful as that of herpes simplex. However, because of the pain and aggravation involved with a shingles outbreak, the essential oils utilized need to be absolutely nonirritant and gentle on the skin.

A blend of Ravintsara (*Cinnamomum camphora*) and Foraha (*Calophyllum inophyllum*) has become the standard treatment option for shingles outbreaks. Especially with elderly patients this treatment almost invariably offers stunning relief from the excruciating pain and brings renewed quality of life. After the initial treatment, frequency and severity of subsequent outbreaks is often reduced drastically. Ravintsara is an antiviral agent and *Calophyllum inophyllum* stimulates phagocytosis (the cellular process of engulfing solid particles by the cell membrane, a major mechanism used to remove pathogens and cell debris).

Influenza

The flu is caused by the influenza virus. Unlike the herpes viruses, which infect skin tissue, the influenza virus invades nasal mucosa, throat, and especially the lungs. Treatment of the flu with essential oils appears to be defined by two aspects. The first is that essential oils are, in fact, effective against the influenza virus. The second is that it is impossible or very difficult to deliver the essential oil to the infected organ tissue where the virus replicates. To counter this disadvantage Pénoël suggests a forceful topical use of essential oils to produce concentrations high enough in the bloodstream to inactivate the virus as it moves from a destroyed cell in search of a new host. Whether this presumed mechanism reflects reality is unclear.

The actual application, however, does produce reasonably successful outcomes. Treatment of the flu with essential oils is not as miraculously effective as the treatment of herpes or even a common cold. Once the influenza virus has infected the lung tissue and the typical symptoms, such as weakness, joint pain, kidney pain, and fever, are all present, simply "cutting off" the infection with a high dosage of essential oils will generally not work. Instead, essential oils are used throughout the duration of the flu to keep the condition contained and prevent secondary bacterial infection.

Without essential oils a secondary bacterial infection of the sinus cavities or the bronchi is common. A simple indicator for its absence is the clear color of eliminated mucus. Colored mucus indicates metabolic debris from bacterial infection.

The aim of the treatment is to stabilize the body during this difficult period and to prevent complications. This may sound moderate, but it has proven to be a reasonable option and, importantly, it avoids the use of antibiotics to treat secondary bacterial infections. By letting the body go through the process, the immune system is given a chance to defeat the virus and will generally emerge strengthened from the episode.

UNDERSTANDING AROMATHERAPY

Shingles Treatment

The classic formula for shingles treatment calls for equal parts of Ravintsara and *Calophyllum inophyllum*. This blend is applied directly onto the lesions. This can be done with a Q-tip or simply by dabbing a few drops onto the lesion with the finger. This is repeated frequently at the beginning of the treatment. (Doing this 4 or 5 times on the first day of treatment is fine.)

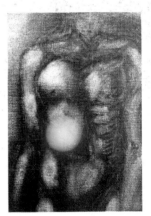

Shingles typically appear on one side (original painting by Monika Haas).

Recipe

Dr. Pam Taylor's Fall-Winter Respiratory Blend

During the fall, winter, and spring, cases of upper respiratory conditions, including influenza, bronchitis, pneumonia, sore throat, and the common cold, are quite frequent. Essential oils quickly reduce symptoms, shorten recovery time, and may be used preventively. Parents often apply this blend to their children before they leave for school and when they come home.

To a blend of 1 part castor oil and 5 parts Jojoba add the following essential oils at 2 drops each per ounce (2 tablespoons/30 ml) of carrier:

Bay	Geranium
Palmarosa	Clove Bud
Benzoin	Sandalwood
Cypress	Thyme
Ginger	Nutmeg
Eucalyptus radiata	Tea Tree
Hyssop decumbens	

The blend can be applied to the throat, upper back, and chest hourly while awake. For infants apply to the bottoms of the feet and on the back to reduce the likelihood of the oil getting on their hands and into their eyes. The homeopathic remedies of Aconite, Bryonia, Gelsemium, and Rhus Tox are particularly useful for influenza; or the Schussler Cell Salts Ferrum Phos and Kali Mur (to relieve cough due to inflammation) may be used where appropriate.

Essential Oils for Common Ailments

Essential Oils for Influenza Treatments

To treat the flu a variety of oils are used. They are selected for their antiviral activity and for being suited for repeated and high-volume application. Consequently, essential oils with high concentrations of stimulating phenols such as Thyme, Oregano, or Savory are generally *not* chosen for flu treatment. Instead, essential oils with equally good antiviral qualities and less propensity to irritate, such as *Eucalyptus radiata* and *Eucalyptus dives,* are employed for frequent topical (rubbing) applications of the torso. Spike Lavender and Thyme thuyanol form another effective combination suited for generous and repeated topical application. Ravintsara is chosen for inhalation and again Spike Lavender and Thyme thuyanol for use in suppositories.

Recent Influenza Viruses: H1N1 Resistance

Due to the media drumbeat about swine flu and the H1N1 virus, awareness of corporate antiviral drugs is on the rise. Almost without exception, reports on the spread of H1N1 mention the drug Tamiflu. (Another drug of the same class, Relenza, is mentioned only rarely.) The uncritical media push of Tamiflu appears odd, given the questionable usefulness of the drug. According to Anthony Fiore, M.D., MPH, and CDC liaison to the influenza working group:

> Oseltamivir-resistant H1N1 is the most commonly isolated virus thus far this season (2009). . . . Clinicians need to know that oseltamivir alone may not effectively prevent or treat influenza. . . . To date, 264 of the tested 268 influenza A H1N1 viruses from the 2008/2009 season were resistant to oseltamivir. Currently, rapid tests to identify influenza A subtypes and antiviral resistance do not exist.[1]

Oseltamivir (the generic name for the active component in Tamiflu) belongs to a class of antiviral drugs that work by specifically inhibiting neuraminidase, which is an enzyme that allows the virus to emerge from a destroyed host cell and to hijack a new cell. Resistance to oseltamivir arises through a minor mutation in the neuraminidase protein: amino acid number 274, histidine, is replaced by tyrosine. Viruses with tyrosine in the 274 position are resistant to oseltamivir. This is a classic example of the drawbacks of monotarget drugs.

Nonselective agents such as essential oils, which interfere with multiple molecular targets, will inactivate viruses regardless of minor changes in the sequence of a specific protein. While essential oils only rarely enjoy verification of their antiviral activities through corporate research, their efficacy is nonetheless well established. A major benefit of essential oil treatment of viral conditions is that due to the nonselective activity of many components, viruses cannot develop resistance.

Tamiflu purportedly reduces the duration of the flu from an average of five or six days by approximately one day. With such modest benefits provided by the corporate drug, essential oil therapy with its proven universal activity appears equally or more effective.

Fungal Infections: Candida and Co.

The antifungal efficacy of essential oils is known experientially and through extensive studies.[2] Yeast infections, caused by *Candida albicans* or similar microorganisms (more correctly referred to as yeast overgrowth syndrome), have become epidemic in Western countries, arguably due to diets rich in refined sugar or similar promoters of candida.

Studies by Pellecuer at the University of Montpellier demonstrated that Mountain Savory oil was highly effective against candida and other yeasts, causing quite a stir in the early 1970s.[3] More recently an interesting twist emerged in the understanding of essential oil efficacy against fungi and yeasts. One of life's key enzymes, HMG CoA reductase (see chapter 1), is not only found in mammals and plants; it is also a key player in the metabolism of yeasts. The enzyme is sensitive to the terpenoid components of essential oils, which effectively shut the enzyme off, ultimately inhibiting the proliferation of the yeast. (For more detail see chapter 13.)

Cystitis

There are similarities in the way our culture labels candidiasis and cystitis as infections, when in reality both conditions are caused by the overgrowth of microorganisms that have always been there. Symptoms associated with both conditions are, at least in part, the result of lifestyle choices. Tea Tree essential oil is classically used for this condition, and it can, according to French aromatherapy, be fortified with a trace of Mountain Savory. Essential oil treatment will ease or eliminate the symptoms in a very short time.

Dr. Pam Taylor on Antibiotic-Resistant Infections

MRSA (multidrug-resistant *Staphylococcus aureus*) is an increasing concern, especially in hospitals, suggesting that bacteria can work around the activity of antibiotics and develop resistance. The rigorous application of the "MRSA Blend" formula has been useful. Frequent application is important—hourly while awake. The patient should also take a good botanical antimicrobial blend frequently, until the condition is resolved. Constitutional hydrotherapies and twice-daily topical applications of an Epsom salt poultice will also speed recovery.

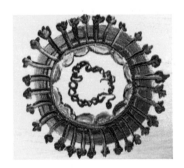

Artist's rendition of a retro virus (original painting by Monika Haas)

Essential Oils for
Common Ailments

Infection or Overgrowth?

Yeast overgrowth is exactly what the term says: it is the opportunistic and sometimes explosive growth of a microorganism as a result of a fertile terrain for its reproduction or the immune system's inability to keep it at bay or both. Yeast overgrowth is typically the consequence of antibiotics or a lifestyle or diet that feeds the yeast.

Essential oil treatments do little to change such lifestyles overnight, but they are very effective in eliminating the overgrowth of yeast and its annoying symptoms.

A blend suggested for treating vaginal or internal yeast could consist of essential oils of Geranium, Marjoram, and possibly a minimal concentration of Cinnamon leaves.

Recipe

MRSA Blend

To each 5 ml (1 teaspoon) of castor oil, 5 ml (1 teaspoon) of *Phytolacca* (Poke Root) oil, and 20 ml (4 teaspoons) of Jojoba, add the following essential oils:

Geranium: 5 drops

Tea Tree: 5 drops

Lavender: 5 drops

Oregano: 5 drops

Thyme: 5 drops

Cassia: 2 drops

Clove Bud: 2 drops

Myrrh: 5 drops

Bay: 4 drops

Depending on the extent and severity of a topical lesion, the following herbal blend may be applied in alternation or substituted as a carrier base.

Antimicrobial Herbal Blend

1 part Echinacea blend (purp. and ang.)

1 part Hypericum

1 part Hydrastis

1 part Propolis

1 part *Populi gemma* (Poplar Bud)

1 part *Usnea barbata*

1 part *Stellaria med.* (Chickweed)

6 parts *Calendula succus*

Allergy Relief

Allergies are learned behavior. The immune system has become sensitized to a certain allergen and will react to renewed exposure to the same allergen with a disproportionate response: an allergic reaction. This is the reason allergies are generally not "curable" overnight. In the best case, they can be undone slowly, by gradually reconditioning the immune system. The two holistic ways to cope with allergies are to avoid the allergen (if known and possible) or to minimize the symptoms.

Two different types of essential oils have been found especially helpful in relieving allergy symptoms. Essential oils from the *Myrtaceae* family such as Tea Tree and Niaouli (*Melaleuca quinquenervia viridiflora* or MQV) have shown antiallergic properties in conventional pharmacological tests. The experience in aromatherapy is that these oils have a noticeable relieving effect when used topically.

The other type of oil with notable antiallergic effects is *Tanacetum annuum* from Morocco. This essential oil, correctly referred to with the vernacular Moroccan Chamomile, contains a large proportion of chamazulene and a variety of sesquiterpene lactones. Through its sesquiterpene lactones, *Tanacetum annuum* modulates the cascade of events that mediate inflammation, ultimately slowing or decreasing the release of histamine.

A classic blend for allergy relief consists of 4.5 ml MQV, 0.5 ml *Tanacetum annuum,* and 3 to 4 drops of Peppermint oil. Allergy symptoms such as runny nose and watery, itchy eyes can be minimized by simply applying 1 or 2 drops of this blend topically on the face. It is advantageous to wash or rinse the face with cold water, simply to create an extra degree of cooling, and then apply the oils on the moist facial skin. While this treatment will not cure the susceptibility to the allergen, it will make the symptoms more bearable. Over time it will contribute to undoing the mistaken conditioning of the immune system.

Another possible aromatherapy approach to reduce allergy symptoms has not yet been sufficiently explored: *Pinus sylvestris* is described in French texts as having cortisone-like qualities and is recognized as a decongestant. The language of Chinese medical aromatherapy agrees, attributing to *Pinus sylvestris* the power to tighten amorphous states in favor of structure. To explore its usefulness the oil could be used topically over the kidney area and possibly as a part of body lotions used to reduce allergic dispositions.

Essential Oils for Common Complaints

Dr. Taylor recommends the use of essential oils in a variety of other circumstances, ranging from easing pain to easing grief.

Pain Relief

The ability to relieve pain is essential. The "Pain Relief Blend" formula has been effective in palliating pain resulting from a wide range of conditions, including Buerger's Disease, fibromyalgia, inflammatory and rheumatoid arthritis, tendonitis, back pain, strains and sprains, carpal tunnel syndrome, and neuritis. There are two components to the formula: a botanical blend of infused oils used as the carrier medium and the essential oils. The blend is applied sparingly and as needed for relief.

The blend may also be used in conjunction with an appropriate homeopathic remedy, for example: Arnica, Calcarea Carbonica, Ruta, Rhus Tox, or Agaricus. For cystitis relief, essential oils of Juniper, Sandalwood, Oregano, and Thyme may be added, along with the daily application of a castor oil pack, until symptoms are relieved.

Recipe

Pain Relief Blend

Carrier Component

1 part *Arnica montana* (infused oil of aerial parts)

1 part Calendula (infused oil of aerial parts)

1 part Hypericum/St. John's Wort (infused oil of aerial parts)

1 part *Ruta graveolens* (infused oil of aerial parts)

1 part Symphytum/Comfrey (infused oil of root and/or aerial parts)

5 parts Jojoba

5 ml/1 teaspoon of castor oil added to each 25 ml of the above blend

Essential Oil Component

To each ounce (2 tablespoons/30 ml) of the above carrier add the following essential oils:

Bay: 2 drops

Helichrysum: 3 drops

Clove Bud: 2 drops

Roman Chamomile: 3 drops

Ginger: 3 drops

Rosemary: 3 drops

Lavender: 3 drops

As with some other recipes from Dr. Taylor, this one calls for a variety of herbal products, some of which may not be readily available. If you cannot locate Calendula infused oil and/or Ruta infused oil, substitute the more readily available St. John's Wort infused oil or simply use more base oil. It is certainly reasonable to use a blend with most of the components instead of not making the remedy at all because some of the components are missing.

Infant Colic

Diet changes are fundamental in resolving infant colic. However, a simple essential oil application can relieve the gas and cramping until these changes are able to take effect. Apply the blend shown in the recipe for infant colic as needed over the abdomen, low back, and bottoms of the feet. If there is a problem with infants getting the oil on their hands and then into their eyes, the application will still be effective when applied to just the back and feet.

Recipe

Infant Colic

To each ounce (2 tablespoons/30 ml) of Jojoba add the following essential oils:

German Chamomile: 2 drops
Lavender: 3 drops
Cardamom: 3 drops
Fennel: 3 drops
Ginger: 3 drops
Peppermint: 2 drops

Insomnia, Shock, and Grief

Essential oils are inherently suited for multiple applications. They add a fundamental element of care to multifocal, family care practice replaceable by no other element.

When I heard that my friend "J" had lost her husband in a horrific car accident, I made her an essential oil "Blend for Shock, Insomnia, and Grief." I suggested she might enjoy applying it to her face and hands. A few weeks later she asked for another bottle. She had found it very effective in resolving a large abdominal ulcer associated with her type 2 diabetes.

Recipe

Blend for Insomnia, Shock, and Grief

To each ounce (2 tablespoons/30 ml) of Jojoba I added 2 drops each of the following essential oils:

Rose	Jasmine
Petitgrain	Neroli
Lavender	Rosewood
Benzoin	Vetiver
Ylang Ylang	

Considerations for the Practicing Therapist

Essential oils offer opportunities for patient care on several levels: acute care, relief in chronic cases, and relief for mental-emotional distress. Their volatile nature and low molecular weight allow them to disperse through the body quickly, generally in less than 2 minutes. They can be applied in the office for acute and chronic conditions, and after a brief period of observation, both the clinician and the patient can determine whether or not the protocol will have a positive effect. Quality is clinically relevant and improved results have been obvious with moving to higher quality essential oils.

Naturopathic physicians are well positioned to understand and make effective clinical use of essential oils. Side effects are rare, generally minimal, and self-limiting, making essential oils a prime illustration of *primum non nocere*, "first do no harm." Essential oils work quickly, safely, and reliably, and they add the benefit of increasing the confidence of both doctor and patient.

Essential oils are cost-effective, portable in a multiple-site practice, lend themselves to custom formulation and dispensing, and take up little office space. Protocols are easy to learn and apply—leading to increased patient compliance and therefore better clinical results. While effective on their own, they also combine well with other protocols, including botanical medicine, diet and nutritional counseling, homeopathy, hydrotherapy, and bodywork.

Essential Oils and Homeopathy

When combining essential oils with homeopathy, check the antidotes for individual remedies. For example: Peppermint will antidote remedies in the Natrum family (Nat. Mur., Nat. Phos., etc.). Chamomile and oils with high camphor content may have an effect on some homeopathic remedies. Otherwise the two protocols should be compatible. As a case in point, Madam Marguerite Maury, using essential oils, and her husband E. A. Maury, M.D., using homeopathic remedies, practiced together to the benefit of their patients.

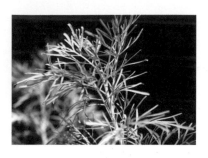

ESSENTIAL OILS AND THE SKIN

The same dynamic effects on cells are obtained at a high dilution.
RENÉ-MAURICE GATTEFOSSÉ, *AROMATHÉRAPIE:
LES HUILES ESSENTIELLES HORMONES VÉGÉTALES*

Skin conditions are particularly responsive to aromatherapy treatments, as the essential oils can be applied directly to the area of the pathological process. Essential oils also appear to have distinct qualities preventing UV damage and melanoma.

Skin Injuries

Helichrysum italicum is so mild that sometimes it is the preferred option for the immediate treatment of injuries, especially bleeding wounds. Dropping this oil into a bleeding wound sanitizes the wound, speeds its closure, and effectively stops the pain. Using it undiluted on wounds avoids bringing other, less suited substances, such as fatty base oils, into the wound. It is self-explanatory that using Helichrysum essential oil on wounds requires a genuine and authentic oil.

Generally, though, the essential oil of *Helichrysum italicum* is best used in dilution (low concentration). For most of its intended purposes it is equally as effective in a 1% dilution in sesame oil as it would be at higher concentrations. Given that the oil is not entirely inexpensive the remarkable efficacy of even the smallest amounts make treatments with *Helichrysum italicum* essential oil quite affordable after all.

Helichrysum and the Skin

The classic example of an essential oil that is highly effective in dilution is *Helichrysum italicum,* the oil that may be aromatherapy's most easily recognizable success story. Its undisputed ability to heal skin tissue steadily increases the demand for this oil. The aromatherapy literature is full of praise and testimonials for this oil. Exploration of this essential oil, also known as Everlasting or Immortelle, offers a nonthreatening experiment. It impresses with its extreme gentleness and high efficacy. There is hardly a better wound healer and antiaging agent than this oil.

To verify this contention, a drop of the essential oil is applied to a random reddish area we may have on our hands or arms, simply to notice the non-event that follows. Either nothing happens or symptoms of irritation diminish or disappear.

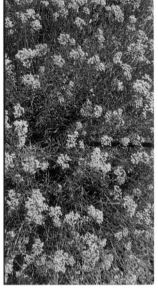

Helichrysum italicum growing in Salagon, France

An Essential Oil with a History

Prior to the war in 1992, large quantities of Helichrysum essential oil were distilled in the former Yugoslavia. Demand came

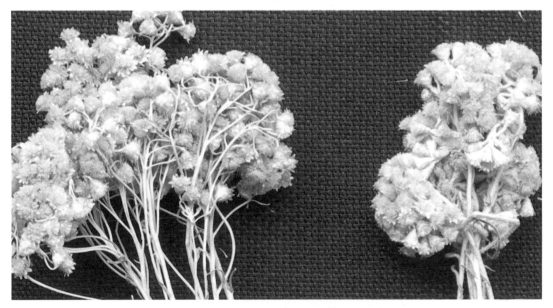

Above left: *Helichrysum italicum* from Corsica
Above right: *Helichrysum italicum* from a hillside in Herzegovina

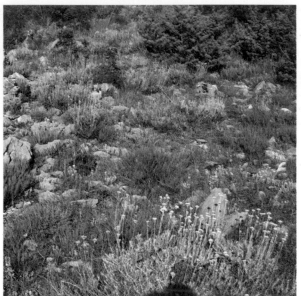

Helichrysum in the wild

mostly from Grasse industries, which employed the oil as an important part in fragrancing/flavoring pipe tobaccos. Aromatherapy was only beginning to discover Helichrysum, and its popularity grew right around the time when the supply from the Balkans dried up due to the war. The only remaining production then came from Corsica, which could not satisfy the demand, and prices began a steady climb.

In the last ten years, production of Helichrysum from the hillsides of Croatia, Bosnia, and Herzegovina has returned to the market. This has not necessarily led to a decrease in prices, as a large multinational corporation has launched a skincare line based on *Helichrysum italicum* essential oil. Helichrysum has remained the subject of a sellers' market.

Oils purportedly originating from mainland France appear to be spurious, as it is illegal to harvest the plant there. Helichrysum oils labeled to be of French (as opposed to Corsican) origin have a higher likelihood of having had at least a minor stay in a laboratory or of being a blend of oils from different growing areas—fabricated in Grasse!

It appears that oils from Corsica and Bosnia-Herzegovina (or other areas of the former Yugoslavia) work equally well for wound and scar treatments, despite the fact they have moderately different chemical composition. Recent analyses have shown very few or no oxygenated components (diketones or molecules with two ketone groups) in some samples of the Bosnian oil. This may be a consequence of harvesting at the earliest possible time, as buyers from France crisscross the growing areas, leaving those who start late with no plants to harvest.

It would be interesting to ascertain whether oxygenated compounds accumulate in Helichrysum oil later rather than earlier in its flowering state. Even though conventional thinking attributes the qualities of Helichrysum essential oil to its content of diketones, the oils with no (or very few) diketones seemingly work equally well. It would appear that the undisputable qualities of this essential oil are better explained by organicism than by identifying active ingredients: the wound-healing quality of Helichrysum oil arises at the level of the whole plant and not at the level of a specific molecule.

> ## Recipe
>
> ### Skin Regeneration with Helichrysum
>
> The classic formula to treat hematomas or bruises calls for 1 part *Helichrysum italicum* oil in 99 parts of a base oil. In other words 1 ml, or roughly 25 drops, of Helichrysum oil can be put in a 4 ounce (or 100 ml) bottle, which is then filled up with the base oil of choice or availability.
>
> To treat old and new scars, cheloids, and stretch marks, the formula is slightly altered to include some Rosehip Seed oil:
>
> 1 ml *Helichrysum italicum* oil and 15 ml Rosehip Seed oil (this can be measured roughly by using an empty 15 ml bottle) are placed in a 4 ounce or 100 ml bottle, which is then filled up with base oil.
>
> The synergy between the omega 3 fatty acids of the Rosehip Seed oil and the terpenoids of the Helichrysum essential oil is fairly miraculous. Even very old scars gradually disappear as this blend is applied to the scar tissue for 1 to 6 months, 2 to 3 times per day.

Eczema

As difficult as it is to find effective answers to this often debilitating condition, searching for solutions with aromatherapy is very much risk free and offers a good potential for success, especially considering that conventional medical thinking has not gone beyond the steroid mantra.

Interestingly, Eastern and Western approaches lead to different suggestions for the treatment of eczema. The language of classical Chinese medicine begins by recognizing the difficulty in treating eczema. It describes the condition as characterized by the simultaneous presence of excess dryness and excess dampness. Western treatment strategies tend to treat one or the other, leading to initial success, but not producing permanent improvement. Chinese medical strategy aims to resolve the presence of two opposing pathogenic factors and suggests harmonizing them rather than treating one aspect or the other. In a purely Chinese perspective, it would be Citrus oils that mediate the harmony between the opposing poles.

Treatment suggestions of French-style aromatherapy also reflect the need for harmony. Oils that firmly hold "the middle" are chosen to regenerate and soothe the skin. The goal is to combine oils that cause

In alignment with more conventional approaches, different types of eczema are distinguished.

Dry Eczema

Two parts of an essential oil component consisting of 2 or 3 tonifying (terpene alcohol rich) essential oils such as Geranium and 2 or 3 skin regenerating (ketone rich) oils like Spike Lavender are combined with 1 part *Calophyllum inophyllum*. This synergy is then worked into an Aloe gel at approximately 2%.

Weeping Eczema

Two parts of an essential oil component consisting of drying oils like Rock Rose (*Cistus ladaniferus*) and regenerating oils such as Rosemary verbenone are combined with one part *Calophyllum*. The synergy is worked into the gel at 2% for topical application.

Eczema with Pustules

In this recipe holistic turns mechanistic: calming *Eucalyptus citriodora* is combined with astringent *Lentiscus pistachius,* liver-regenerating Thyme thuyanol, and lymph-supporting *Laurus nobilis*. Two parts essential oil blend are combined with 1 part *Calophyllum* in the usual fashion.

little or no physical sensation but still regenerate and normalize the skin. At the same time, kidney function, crucial for clearing conditions such as eczema, should be supported. Oils meeting these criteria are St. John's Wort, *Solidago canadiensis, Abies balsamea,* and *Picea mariana.* This synergy represents a starting point that can easily be modified according to preference or specific conditions.

Recipe

Symptomatic Relief for Eczema and Psoriasis

The following formula has been effective for symptomatic relief until the underlying cause can be corrected.

To each 4 ounces of Carlson vitamin E cream add the following essential oils:

Bay: 4 drops
Lavender: 20 drops
Carrot Seed: 5 drops
Geranium: 5 drops

With the addition of 5 ml (1 teaspoon) of castor oil, this blend can also help reduce scar tissue, minor burns, insect bites, and stings. It provides symptomatic relief of poison ivy and for small cuts and abrasions. With the addition of 5 ml (1 teaspoon) of the Antimicrobial Herbal Blend (see page 146) per 4 ounces of vitamin E cream, it is very effective in controlling acne. (Recipe by Pam Taylor)

Psoriasis

Conventional medical language states that the exact causes of psoriasis are not known. Phrases found on the Internet culminate in: "Psoriasis is a puzzle." The absence of an immune system response to psoriasis suggests that it is not caused by outside factors but is instead an aberration of our own (skin) metabolism.

Essential oil treatment aims to rectify virtually every skin problem. The main agent to do so is *Nardostachys jatamansii* or Spikenard. This oil was originally recommended by Dietrich Gümbel, the pioneer of an anthroposophical approach to skin care, to rectify virtually every skin problem.[1] *Nardostachys jatamansii* essential oil is extremely well tolerated and regenerates the skin most gently. The original impulse to use this oil for skin treatments most likely arose from the anthroposophical fascination with plants with an open, in other words eternal, life cycle.

Spikenard can be complemented by minute quantities of Mountain Savory with its forceful reanimating components, Niaouli (*Melaleuca quinquenervia viridiflora* or MQV) with its unrivaled restorative powers, and *Lippia citriodora,* which balances nervous and endocrine systems.

Jimm Harrison on the Prevention of UV Damage and Melanoma

The antioxidant and anti-inflammatory properties of essential oils have been recognized for their ability to protect from photoaging (damage that is done to the skin from prolonged exposure to UV radiation). Yet they have drawn little attention for their ability to prevent skin cancer. Jimm Harrison has extensively researched the combination of essential oils with other natural substances useful for regenerative skin care. The following review of their efficacy for prevention of sun damage was originally presented by him at the 7th Scientific Aromatherapy Conference in San Francisco, February 2009.

Sandalwood Oil

Sandalwood oil was used topically for twenty weeks and was found to decrease the incidence of skin papillomas. It inhibited 12-O-tetra-decanoylphorbol-13-acetate (TPA) induced epidermal ornithine decarboxylase (ODC) activity. The latter process is a prominent or marker event in skin cancer and used to study substances for their preventative capacity. The study implicated alpha-santalol as the active compound.

Eugenol

4-Allyl-2-methoxyphenol (eugenol), a component of Clove (*Eugenia caryophyllata*) essential oil, was found to be a potent inhibitor of melanoma cell proliferation. Eugenol produced a significant tumor-growth delay and an almost 40 percent decrease in tumor size and was well tolerated, as determined by measurement of body weights. Examination of the mechanism of the antiproliferative action of eugenol in the human malignant melanoma cell line showed that it arrests cells in the S phase of the cell cycle.

Recipe

Formulation Suggestions for Topical Applications to Prevent Sun Damage

The easiest formula to concoct is a simple blend of fixed oils and essential oils.

Fixed Oils
> Olive oil 30–70%
> Sunflower seed oil 30–70%
> Cranberry seed oil 3–10%

Essential Oil Complex 2–5%

The essential oils are given below in the order of suggested higher to lower concentration:
> Palmarosa
> Lavender
> Copaiba
> Clove
> Frankincense

Nourishing Components
> Rosehip Seed CO_2 0.5%–2%
> D-alpha-tocopherol 1–2%

Frankincense

Antitumor and chemopreventive effects were shown for alpha- and beta-boswellic acid acetate isolated from *Boswellia carterii.* The authors concluded that it would be useful in prevention of primary tumor invasion and metastasis. Several studies have documented the chemopreventive effects of boswellic acid on a variety of cancer cells. In a treatment study the whole essential oil of Frankincense was used on a horse with multicentric malignant melanoma. The oil was injected directly into the tumors and also applied topically. In biopsies following the treatment it was demonstrated that "small tumor" cells were destroyed by the injected Frankincense essential oil while the tumors treated topically were reduced in size.

Thyme and Carvacrol

A patient with AJCC (American Joint Committee on Cancer) stage III melanoma, refusing the proposed treatment, used ground leaves and stems of Thyme (*Thymus vulgaris*) in an herbal tea and for topical applications in compresses over the lesions. There was a progressive disappearance of all nodules over the period of a few weeks and a confirmed complete regression of cutaneous metastases. A follow-up with the patient showed no evidence of disease after five years. As reported in the *Journal of the American Academy of Dermatology,* the authors were noncommittal as to the regression being due to the use of Thyme extract, though pointed out a chronological relationship between the use of Thyme and regression.

Thyme extract, as used by the patient, was an infusion, making it difficult to assume that the essential oil alone would have a similar effect. There are other studies that support the antitumor activity of Thyme essential oil. The essential oil of *Thymus broussonettii,* containing carvacrol (83.18 percent), along with paracymene, gamma-terpinene, and transcaryophyllene, was shown to have antitumor effect.

There are many species of Thyme and various chemotypes. The results of a study using eleven Moroccan Thyme essential oils showed that all had important cytotoxic effects, with carvacrol being the most cytotoxic compound. Carvacrol, in an alternate study, was also shown to be a very potent inhibitor of cell growth in human non–small cell lung cancer cell line (A549). Thymol has demonstrated cytotoxicity on human leukemic K562 cells. In all studies the compounds and oils showed no cytotoxicity to healthy cells.

Chemoprevention by Polyphenolic Compounds, Flavonoids, and Carotenoids

It's well documented that a diet of vegetables, fruit, and herbs rich in flavonoids, carotenoids, and polyphenolic components will help to protect the body and skin from damage by UV exposure, including skin cancers, melanoma, photoaging, and hyperpigmentation. Dietary recommendations thus include high amounts of "colored" foods, which have been well researched for their antioxidant activity and potential to prevent and reverse cancers. However, the amount of the compounds found within the beneficial foods necessary for complete protection may exceed what is consumed even in the healthiest diet. Supplementation seems to be a sensible approach to enhance the benefits of these nutrients.

Flavonoids for UV-Related Skin Damage

Different groups of flavonoids (a class of secondary metabolites or yellow pigments) are distinguished: flavanes, flavanones, flavones, flavonols, catechines, anthocyanidins, and isoflavone. They all have common antioxidant, anti-inflammatory, antitumor, antiviral, and antibacterial properties, as well as a direct cytoprotective effect on coronary and vascular systems, the pancreas, and the liver. There are many studies that demonstrate the actions of flavonoids on melanoma cells.

Carotenoids

Carotenoids represent one of the more popular subjects in nutritional sciences. These lipophilic, photosynthetic pigments in plants are prod-

Recipe

A Suggested Fatty Oil/Essential Oil//Nutrient/Tincture Formula

Fatty Oil Blend

    Olive oil 15–40%

    Sesame oil 10–30%

    Sunflower seed oil 15–40%

    Rosehip Seed oil 2–10%

    Cranberry seed oil 2–10%

    Shea butter 5–20%

    Cocoa butter 5–15%

Essential Oil Complex 2–5%

The essential oils are given below in the order of suggested higher to lower concentration:

    Rosemary verbenone

    Copaiba

    Frankincense

    Helichrysum italicum

    Angelica

    Artemisia douglasiana

    Clove

    Myrrh

Tincture Component

    Arnica tincture 2–5%

    Green Tea extract 2–5%

    Sea Buckthorn CO_2 0.5–1%

    Rosehip Seed CO_2 0.5–1%

    Tocotrienol mix 1–2%

    D-alpha-tocopherol 1%

    Alpha lipoic acid 0.25%

    MSM 1–2%

    Ascorbyl palmitate 1%

ucts of the terpenoid biosynthetic pathway. They are well studied for the treatment and prevention of skin cancer and UV-related skin damage. The carotenoids beta-carotene and astaxanthin have also been shown to protect against sunburn through internal supplementation.

Resveratrol

Resveratrol is a natural phenol from a class of compounds called stilbenes found in grape skin, red wine, peanuts, and berries. Interest in resveratrol was heightened by the "French Paradox," the surprisingly low incidence of heart disease in populations who consume diets high in saturated fats and red wine.

Green Tea Polyphenols (-)-Epigallocatechin-3-gallate

Green Tea (*Camellia sinensis*) contains potent antioxidants and is known to protect genes and cells from oxidative damage. Epidemiological observations have shown very low rates of cancer in Green-Tea consuming countries. A study was performed to see if the results demonstrating that Green Tea polyphenols (GTP) reduced the risk for skin cancer in a murine photocarcinogenesis model could also be observed in human cells.

Ginger

[6]-Gingerol of fresh Ginger (*Zingiber officinalis*) has antioxidant, apoptotic, and anti-inflammatory properties; it was also found to provide protection against UVB-induced skin disorders. As there is a correlation between malignant melanomas and COX-2 expression, [6]-Gingerol is apparently chemopreventive, for it suppresses NF-kappa beta, the essential transcription factor responsible for the release of COX-2. Other components in Ginger such as vallinoids, [6]-paradol, shogaols, and zingerone have also been studied and found to have chemopreventive effects.

Turmeric

Curcumin is extracted from Turmeric (*Curcuma longa*) and known as the Indian curry spice. It has been used in treatment of squamous cell carcinoma and melanoma, as well as many other forms of cancer, with actions that may be explained by its ability to interfere with multiple cell signaling pathways.

Pomegranate Seed Oil

In an experiment to determine chemopreventive efficacy of pomegranate (*Punica granatum*) seed oil in mice, it was found to be an agent against skin cancer. The major components found in pomegranate seed oil—anthocyanins, ellagitannins, and hydrolyzable tannins—are phenolic antioxidants that exhibit very strong radical scavenging effects.

Fatty Oils

Olive Oil

Topical treatment with extra virgin olive oil (*Olea europa*) reduced UVB-induced skin tumors in mice.

Polyunsaturated and Other Fatty Acids

In several studies, fatty acids extracted from vegetables and fruit were used to decrease the number of melanoma cells. Results showed arachidonic and linoleic acids most effective in decreasing S91 murine melanoma cells; palmitic acid was most toxic toward B16F10 murine melanoma cells.

Omega-3 fatty acids are most effective against melanoma. Docosahexaenoic acid (DHA), an omega-3 polyunsaturated fatty acid, inhibits the proliferation of human metastatic melanoma cells. Studies using fish oils, rich in omega-3 fatty acids, demonstrate the protective benefits against UVR damage with dietary supplementation.

Sesame and Sunflower: Sesamol

Sesame (*Sesamum indicum*) seed has been recognized as a potent healing agent especially within Ayurvedic practice. Certain fatty acids in sesame, including linoleic acid and oleic acid, are known for their anti-carcinogenic effects and cytotoxicity to melanoma cells. An evaluation of the effects of sesamol, found in sesame seed and sunflower seed oils, has shown remarkable chemopreventive effects as well as profound free radical scavenging activity. The study showed sesamol to reduce mouse skin papillomas by 50 percent.

TWELVE

TREATING CHEMOTHERAPY-INDUCED VOMITING AND NAUSEA

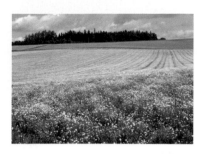

We do not destroy the land because the land is where the herbs are to help us to cure people.

TOMAS AGUILAR,
IN *SHADOWCATCHERS* BY STEVE WALL

This chapter presents Dr. Pam Taylor's recommended uses of essential oils to ease the side effects of chemotherapy, particularly chemotherapy-induced vomiting and nausea (CINV),[1] which occur in 30 to 90 percent of patients undergoing treatment, depending on the chemotherapy drugs used. Symptoms can be so persistent and severe that patients may limit or even forego treatment. Her recommendations are specifically for the layperson who wants to care for a friend or family member undergoing conventional cancer treatment. In other words, Dr. Taylor lends the authority of the practicing naturopathic physician to the instructions for simple aromatherapy remedies, which put the nonprofessional in a position to provide simple but effective help for those in need.

Stages of CINV

Acute CINV occurs in the first twenty-four hours after chemotherapy. Delayed CINV occurs after the first twenty-four hours, lasting up to ninety-six hours. Patients also develop CINV as a learned or a conditioned response when nausea and vomiting during previous treatments was not well controlled. Breaking the reflex/response cycle can prevent or reduce symptoms. This may be accomplished at several points in symptom development through the use of essential oils.

According to Taylor, topical application and inhalation of essential oils can be effective, especially when patients are too nauseated to ingest anything. Essential oils or essential oil blends can be applied directly over the affected area to help relax muscle spasms, over the stomach and back of the neck to relieve nausea, or over the abdomen and lower back to relieve cramping and colic. Essential oils spread through the body rapidly and offer quick relief even with this indirect method of application. When beginning an essential oil support regimen for CINV, it is important to start with small amounts of essential oils and to work within the limits of each individual's tolerance and comfort.

It is important to remember that essential oils are eliminated quickly. If the nausea and vomiting are severe or persistent, essential oils should therefore be reapplied frequently, to maintain the beneficial effect and prevent a reoccurrence of the discomfort.

The Nausea and Vomiting Pathway

The chemoreceptor trigger zone (CTZ) and vomiting center lie near one another in the medulla, the lower part of the brain stem connecting the spinal cord to the cerebellum, a region of the brain that plays an important role in motor control. Stimulation of the CTZ triggers a nerve impulse along the fifth, seventh, tenth, and twelfth cranial nerves to the stomach and muscles of the diaphragm and abdomen, resulting in reverse peristalsis (vomiting). Nausea is an awareness of the stimulation of the vomiting center.

Chemotherapeutic drugs stimulate chemoreceptors in the brain and the digestive tract, including receptors that respond to the neurotransmitter acetylcholine. Inhibiting the uptake of acetylcholine helps prevent the stimulation of the receptor sites involved in chemotherapeutically-induced nausea and vomiting (CINV). Reducing or inhibiting spasms of the stomach and intestines will also prevent or lessen the frequency of vomiting.

Chemotherapy drugs and radiation treatments also cause vomiting

UNDERSTANDING AROMATHERAPY

Essential Oils to Relieve Nausea by Inhibiting Acetylcholine

Lavender (*Lavandula angustifolia, x intermedia, latifolia, Lavender* spp.)
Rosemary (*Rosmarinus off.*)
Frankincense (*Boswellia carterii*)
Scots Pine (*Pinus sylvestris*)
Sweet Marjoram (*Origanum majorana*)
Ylang Ylang (*Cananga odorata*)
Juniper (*Juniperus communis*)

Treating Chemotherapy-Induced Vomiting and Nausea

by triggering the release of serotonin from the mucous membrane lining of the gut, which activates peripheral and afferent nerves.

Conventional Antinausea Agents

Conventional medicine attempts to control CINV with more drugs, including: phenothiazines (chlorpromazine), corticosteroids, haloperidol and droperidol (dopamine 2 or D2 antagonists, which affect motor control), and serotonin type 3 receptor antagonists and NK-1 receptor antagonists (which reduce contractions of the abdominal muscles).

Efficacy of Essential Oils in CINV

Essential oils can reduce or relieve nausea and vomiting by inhibiting acetylcholine, thus avoiding the unwanted and unpleasant side effects of conventional medications. They can be used for controlling CINV in the following ways:

1. To relieve the side effects of conventional medications
2. As primary agents of relief
3. To reduce dosage levels of conventional drugs
4. To break the reflex-response cycle

To be useful for controlling the symptoms of CINV, essential oils should have one or more of the following qualities: antispasmodic, carminative, calming, sedative, and nervine.

- Antispasmodic essential oils include Ginger, Peppermint, and Chamomile.
- Carminative essential oils help reduce or prevent the formation of intestinal gas. Examples include Cardamom, Chamomile, Ginger, Peppermint, Fennel, and Cinnamon.
- Essential oils that are calming, sedative, and tonic to the nervous system include Chamomile, Lavender, Lemon, Rosewood, and Vetiver.

The following essential oils are particularly suited to aid the digestive tract of cancer patients.

Cardamom (*Elettaria cardamomum*)

Cardamom contains the acetylcholine antagonist borneol, which is important in disrupting the pathways that trigger nausea and vomiting. It prevents the formation of intestinal gas, reduces pain, has a relaxing effect, particularly on a spasmodic colon, stimulates the digestive activities of the stomach, and has an expectorant action on the bronchi and lungs. It is useful in relieving painful diarrhea.

Like most essential oils, Cardamom is protective against infection, showing an inhibitory effect on *Staphylococcus aureus, E. Coli,* and *Candida albicans.*

German Chamomile (*Chamomila recutita*)

Chamomile is anti-inflammatory: it inhibits the arachidonic acid pathway, which produces the prostaglandins that mediate inflammation and pain. Chamazulene inhibits inflammation and apigenine, an antioxidant bioflavonoid, scavenges free radicals. Alpha bisabolol provides antispasmodic properties and helps prevent the formation of ulcers.

As a digestive tonic, Chamomile relieves cramping and colicky pains, prevents or reduces the formation of intestinal gas, heals the tissues of an inflamed gut or ulcer, and reduces scar tissue. On the emotional plane it has a universal calming effect. Chamomile reduces mast cell degranulation, preventing the release of histamine and thereby reducing inflammation and common allergic symptoms.

Chamomile is antipyretic, antiseptic, and antibacterial against *Streptococcus pyogenes,* an organism that can cause sore throat, impetigo, erysipelas, cellulite, necrotizing fasciitis, toxic shock syndrome, and myositis (inflammation of the muscles). Chamomile is also active against *Staphylococcus aureus, Bacillus subtilis,* and fungal infections.

Ginger (*Zingiber officinalis*)

Being members of the *Zingiberaceae* family, Ginger and Cardamom share similar healing characteristics. Ginger inhibits COX-2 and other endogenous mediators of inflammation, effectively relieving pain and reducing inflammation. It prevents intestinal gas formation, stimulates the digestive functions of the stomach, suppresses coughs, and has an expectorant action on the bronchi and lungs. It relieves symptoms of fatigue. An effective antispasmodic, Ginger also reduces fevers while

German Chamomile Contraindications

There are no known contraindications for German Chamomile. In rare cases, some individuals may have a reaction, generally a skin rash. This is also true of Roman Chamomile (*Anthemis nobilis*). Allergic reactions to Chamomile are a disputed issue. If and when irritation claimed to have been caused by Chamomile is investigated more closely, it is invariably revealed that other factors are the cause of the irritation. This is made even more prevalent through the preponderance of industrially manipulated Chamomile oils!

Treating Chemotherapy-Induced Vomiting and Nausea

Ginger Contraindications

Because Ginger decreases platelet aggregation (i.e., makes the formation of blood clots less likely), it should be used cautiously in patients who are on blood thinners, whose skin and blood vessels are fragile due to long-term steroid use, hemophiliacs, or those who have other bleeding disorders. Lab tests for coagulation will indicate if adding Ginger to the treatment protocol is becoming problematic. Also look for signs of easy bruising, or petechiae: small, red areas in the skin indicating ruptured capillaries.

Lemon Cautionary Note

Essential oil of Lemon may cause photosensitivity when its use is combined with prolonged exposure to the sun. It can cause some vasoconstriction in the kidneys, so caution may be advised when kidney function is compromised.

promoting perspiration. Its action is gentle, making it appropriate for children as well as the elderly.

In the cardiovascular system, Ginger decreases platelet aggregation to help reduce the risk of blood clots (see sidebar for contraindications). It is inotropic to the heart, helping to normalize the rate at which the heart beats by regulating heart muscle contractility. Ginger helps to relieve symptoms of CINV, as well as nausea and vomiting after surgery. As a choleretic, it stimulates the production of bile in the liver. It is hypolipidemic, helping to lower cholesterol and triglycerides. It can inhibit the development of ulcers in the digestive tract.

Ginger is antimicrobial, diuretic, analgesic, antioxidant, and helps reduce the frequency and severity of migraines. Perhaps more importantly for those receiving chemotherapy or radiation, Ginger stimulates Phase II detoxification pathways to offset oxidative damage in the liver and lungs and relieve the xenobiotic load on the body.

Lavender (*Lavandula angustifolia*)

Lavender is anti-inflammatory, analgesic, antispasmodic, and dispels intestinal gas. It is healing to damaged skin and intestinal tissues, and will resolve scars and burns. It is active against *Staphylococcus aureus, Diplococcus pneumoniae, E. coli, Beta-hemolytic strep.,* and *Klebsiella,* among others. Lavender is also antifungal, making it effective against *Candida albicans* and athlete's foot.

As a muscle relaxant, it helps reduce hypertension (high blood pressure) and tachycardia (a normal heart rate is around 80 beats per minute; tachycardia is an abnormally rapid heart rate of over 100 beats per minute). Its anticoagulant effect is mild. Lavender is anxiolytic and useful in dealing with insomnia. Along with Chamomile, it can relieve a spasmodic cough.

Lemon (*Citrus limon*)

Essential oil of Lemon has a calming and, like other Citrus oils, an antidepressant effect. It dispels intestinal gas, has a stimulant and tonic effect on the digestive system, is antispasmodic, and aids expectoration.

Lemon is antibacterial, antiseptic, and strongly antiviral due to its limonene content. In the cardiovascular system it reduces capillary permeability, thereby preventing easy bruising and bleeding. It is a hypotensive aid to reducing blood pressure. Along with Lavender and

Ginger: Distillation vs. CO$_2$ Extract

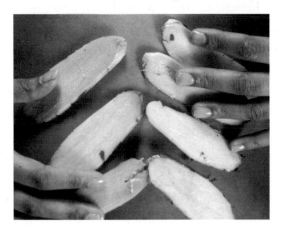

Sliced Ginger root

Ginger is described as an effective carminative and sexual tonic. Its oil is in the underground stem of the plant. Much of its fragrance is due to the essential oil, but its pungent taste is caused by nonvolatile phenylpropanoid derivatives of the gingerol and shogaol moiety.

According to the ISO (International Organization for Standardization) norms, essential oils are steam distilled or cold pressed. Nonetheless carbon dioxide extracts of aromatic plants have become increasingly popular. CO$_2$ extract and steam-distilled essential oils of the same plant species generally have a different chemical composition, reflecting the difference in the production process. Steam distillation requires the aromatic molecules to evaporate, whereas CO$_2$ extraction involves dissolving them in the extraction liquid, in this case supercritical carbon dioxide. CO$_2$ will extract the same lipophilic components that appear in an essential oil. In addition, more polar water-soluble components not found in the essential oil will be extracted.

Ginger is a perfect illustration for this phenomenon. The sharp principals of Ginger, the shogaols and gingerols, are only found in the CO$_2$ extract and give it a stinging quality. The CO$_2$ extract is best used as a component in blends. The steam-distilled essential oil, on the other hand, is warm, gentle, and soft, without the sharp components. It is better suited for topical application than the CO$_2$ extract.

Ginger Candy from Macau is an exquisite specialty. Even visitors from nearby Hong Kong stock up on these candies when they visit the gambling paradise.

Chamomile, it is useful in cases of insomnia. Lemon is also tonic to the liver and kidneys, helping to decongest the tissues.

Peppermint (*Mentha x piperita*)

Peppermint relieves pain, prevents the formation of intestinal gas, breaks up mucus and relieves sinus congestion, and relieves or reduces symptoms of nausea and vomiting. It is antispasmodic (due to the effect of menthol on calcium in the body), choleretic, cholagogic (promoting the flow of bile from the gallbladder into the duodenum), carminative, disinfectant, analgesic, and diaphoretic (promoting increased perspiration).

These combined properties of Peppermint are what make it so effective in relieving nausea, vomiting, flatulence, and spasmodic contractions of the muscles in the digestive tract. It is also tonic to the liver, heart, stomach, and pancreas. Peppermint tends to be mentally stimulating, with an antidepressant effect.

Peppermint is antiviral, antimalarial, antifungal, and generally anti-infectious. It acts specifically against *Bacillus subtilis, Candida albicans, Diplococcus pneumoniae, E. coli, Beta-hemolytic streptococcus, Klebsiella, Mycobacterium tuberculosis, Proteus, Pseudomonas aeruginosa,* and *Staphylococcus aureus,* among others.

Because Peppermint's effects are strong, use small amounts. For example, in a blend for infants and children up to seven years old, and the frail elderly, 1 or 2 drops per ounce (2 tablespoons/30 ml) of carrier base is sufficient. In a blend for older children and adults, use 2 to 3 drops per ounce of carrier base.

UNDERSTANDING AROMATHERAPY

Peppermint Contraindications

Care must be taken if a hiatal hernia is present as Peppermint may cause increased relaxation of the esophageal sphincter and aggravate a tendency toward reflux (GERD).

Peppermint and other herbs and essential oils that are emmenagogues (which stimulate or increase menstrual flow) are traditionally used in much smaller doses and generally have little or no side effects. However, there has been concern by herbalists and aromatherapists (in the U.S.) that Peppermint not be used during pregnancy for fear of its emmenagogue quality (a thought that seems overcautious to the author, P. Taylor). In any case, consultation with a medical herbalist or aromatherapist is recommended before using an emmenagogue during pregnancy.

European practitioners distinguish between emmenagogues—herbs or essential oils that will bring on an otherwise normal (but delayed) menstruation—and abortifacients—herbs that have the potential to cause a pregnant woman to abort a fetus. Herbs and essential oils capable of causing an abortion have potentially severe toxic side effects, partly because they must be used in large doses to achieve an abortion. Such use of an abortifacient can seriously injure vital organs, sometimes resulting in the death of mother and unborn child. As well as being dangerous, abortifacient herbs are unreliable in their effect.

Peppermint can antidote some homeopathic remedies, mainly those in the Natrum family (Nat. Mur, Nat. Phos, Nat. Sulph, etc.). Check with a trained homeopath before using this essential oil if the individual is using homeopathy. In general, the concurrent use of well-chosen essential oils and well-chosen homeopathic remedies is not problematic.

Versatile Efficacy of Essential Oils for Healing the Skin

Essential oils can also be used to alleviate radiation burns, another of the side effects of conventional cancer treatment. The idea, as with many of Dr. Taylor's recommendations, is to give the layperson a simple formula that can be easily adapted to what is available at a specific moment.

> ### Recipe
>
> #### Sample Formula for Skin Healing, Scar Reduction, and Relief from Radiation Burn
>
> To 4 ounces of Carlson vitamin E cream add:
>
> 5 ml/1 teaspoon castor oil
> 5 ml/1 teaspoon *Calophyllum inophyllum* (optional)
> 5 ml/1 teaspoon *Calendula succus*
> 20 drops Lavender
> 10 drops Geranium
> 5 drops Helichrysum (optional)
> 5 drops Frankincense (optional)
> 4 drops Bay
> 4 drops Carrot Seed (optional)
>
> Apply sparingly and frequently (4 to 6 times a day) to affected area.

Treating Chemotherapy-
Induced Vomiting and Nausea

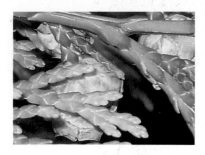

THIRTEEN

AROMATHERAPY AND CANCER

If the scientists continue like this, humanity will die of hunger amidst abundant food.

ARTHUR HERMES

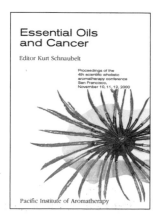

Cancer is probably more feared than any other condition. Attempts by science to find a cure have produced some results, but the progress has not taken the fear away. Until recently, there has not been enough opportunity to verify the usefulness of essential oils in connection with cancer treatments. However, the erstwhile suspicion that essential oils are of help has now been confirmed.

Essential Oils and Cancer: The Beginning

Despite no one in corporate pharmacology paying attention, highly significant academic research in the 1990s focused on the antitumor activity of terpenoid essential oil components. Perillyl alcohol, a terpene alcohol closely related to limonene, was tested in clinical trials for its efficacy against mammary cancer. A key patent claiming cancer treatments with terpenoids is in the possession of the United States. PIA conducted a symposium "Essential Oils and Cancer" in the year 2000, where Charles Elson and Dennis Peffley, two of the most important contributors to the NIH sponsored research, presented their results.

The most immediately applicable result of their work was that a diet rich in mixed and varied terpenoids, that is, a diet rich in fruits and vegetables, verifiably lowered cancer risk. Equally interesting was

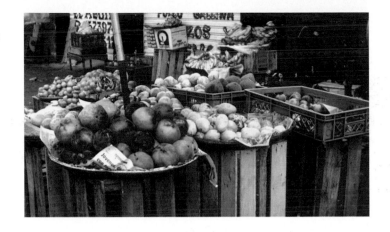

Western science confirms what Grandma said: A diet rich in fruits and vegetables has been found to be the only effective way to significantly reduce cancer risk!

that this dietary approach was the only factor that, over the years, truly reduced cancer risk. Other measures advocated by the supplement industry, such as excess intake of Vitamin E or carotene, were recognized as ineffective.

Sterol Insensitive HMG CoA Reductase

Essential oils can inhibit tumors by multiple mechanisms. One investigated by Elson and Peffley, involving HMG CoA reductase, shall be briefly outlined here. To understand this mechanism it is necessary to recognize the crucial importance of cholesterol for cell membranes. Cholesterol is a three-dimensional molecule—a steroid—that derives rigidity from its specific molecular structure. Rigid cholesterol molecules are inserted into the fluid bilayer cell membrane for added stability. This rigidity is the contribution of cholesterol to a functioning cell membrane. Without cholesterol new cells cannot form and without new cells there is no tissue regeneration.

Under normal metabolic conditions, the production of cholesterol stops once there is sufficient cholesterol available. In a typical feedback loop, excess cholesterol tells the HMG CoA reductase enzyme to stop the synthesis once there is enough. In cell biology jargon the enzyme is said to be "sterol sensitive." It switches off once there is enough cholesterol.

The relevance of this mechanism appeared to Elson and Peffley when they noticed a crucial coincidence: that the HMG CoA reductase of tumor cells differs from that of healthy cells, but resembles that of fungi. To better understand, let us look at fungi for a moment. In fungi, HMG CoA reductase works the same as in all other organisms—it produces steroids for membrane stability—but it does so with a slight

Aromatherapy and Cancer

Patents on Terpenes

This is the cover of a patent held by the United States on "Monoterpenes, Sesquiterpenes and Diterpenes in Cancer Therapy."[1] Such patents are written in broad generalizing language to include many possibilities, so the mere fact that this patent exists does not necessarily mean that any of the stated therapeutic proposals ultimately would work, especially as this patent was written early in the sequence of research events. However, the clinical trials that followed were considered to be very successful. The respective research is easily looked up online, but by the year 2002 there were almost no more documents about research in this field.

US005602184A

United States Patent [19]

Myers et al.

[11] Patent Number: 5,602,184

[45] Date of Patent: Feb. 11, 1997

[54] **MONOTERPENES, SESQUITERPENES AND DITERPENES AS CANCER THERAPY**

[75] Inventors: **Charles E. Myers**, Rockville; **Jane Trepel**, Bethesda; **Edward Sausville**, Silver Spring; **Dvorit Samid**, Rockville; **Alexandra Miller**, Hyattsville; **Gregory Curt**, Rockville, all of Md.

[73] Assignee: **The United States of America as represented by Department of Health and Human Services**, Washington, D.C.

[21] Appl. No.: **25,471**

[22] Filed: **Mar. 3, 1993**

[51] Int. Cl.^{6} H61K 31/045
[52] U.S. Cl. 514/739
[58] Field of Search 514/739

[56] **References Cited**

U.S. PATENT DOCUMENTS

5,243,094 9/1993 Borg 568/822

FOREIGN PATENT DOCUMENTS

0285302	10/1988	European Pat. Off. .
0393973	10/1990	European Pat. Off. .
2270544	11/1987	Japan .
3098562	4/1991	Japan .
9218465	10/1992	WIPO .

OTHER PUBLICATIONS

Crowell, P. L., et al., "Human metabolism of orally administered d–limonene," *Proc. Amer. Assoc. Cancer Res.*, vol. 33, p. 524, No. 3134 (Mar. 1992).

Crowell, P. L., et al., "Selective Inhibition of Isoprenylation of 21–26–kDa Proteins by the Anticarcinogen d–Limonene and Its Metabolites," *J. Biol. Chem.* 266(26):17679–17685 (Sep. 15, 1991).

Elegbede, J. A., et al., "Regression of Rat Primary Mammary Tumors Following Dietary d–Limonene," *JNCI* 76(2):323–325 (Feb. 1986).

Wattenberg. L. W., et al., "Inhibition of 4–(methylnitrosamino)–1–(3–pyridyl)–1–butanone carcinogenesis in mice by D–limonene and citrus fruit oils," *Carcinogenesis* 12(1):115–117 (1991).

"d–Limonene, an Anticarcinogenic Terpene," *Nutrition Reviews* 46(10):363–365 (Oct. 1988).

Elson, C. E., et al., "Anti–carcinogenic activity of d–limonene during the initiation and promotion/progression stages of DMBA–induced rat mammary carcinogenesis," *Carcinogenesis* 9(2):331–332 (1988).

Webb, D. R., et al., "Assessment of the Subchronic Oral Toxicity of d–Limonene in Dogs," *Fd Chem. Toxic* 28(10):669–675 (1990).

Maltzman, T. R. et al., "The prevention of nitrosomethy–lurea–induced mammary tumors by d–limonene and orange oil," *Carcinogenesis* 10(4):781–783 (19890.

Carter, B. S., et al., "*ras* Gene Mutations in Human Prostate Cancer," *Cancer Research* 50:6830–3832 (Nov. 1, 1990).

Isaacs, W. B., et al., "Genetic Changes Associated with Prostate Cancer in Humans," *Cancer Surveys* vol. 11 (Prostate Cancer), 15–24 (1991).

Casey, P. J., et al., "p21ras is modified by a farnesyl isoprenoid," *Proc. Natl. Acad. Sci. USA* 86:8323–8327 (Nov., 1989).

Primary Examiner—Jerome D. Goldberg
Attorney, Agent, or Firm—Townsend and Townsend and Crew LLP

[57] **ABSTRACT**

The invention provides methods of treating cancer including administering an effective amount of selected terpenes to a mammal having the cancer when the cancer is prostate cancer, colon cancer, astrocytoma, or sarcoma. The terpene is selected from the group consisting of a cyclic monoterpene, a noncyclic monoterpene, a noncyclic sesquiterpene and a noncyclic diterpene. The invention also provides a method of sensitizing a cancer to radiation including administering an effective amount of a terpene to a mammal having the cancer wherein the terpene is selected from the group noted above. Additionally, the invention provides methods of inhibiting the growth of cancer cells including applying an effective amount of a selected terpene to the cancer cells which are cells of prostate cancer, colon cancer, osteosarcoma, or glioblastoma.

19 Claims, 13 Drawing Sheets

difference. Since fungal organisms often colonize their host with explosive growth, they have learned to generate massive amounts of new cells, literally overnight. As a result, switching off the synthesis of the membrane-stabilizing steroids (such as cholesterol) that are needed for new cells is not an issue. Instead, more is better. This may be among the reasons why fungal HMG CoA reductase—otherwise extremely similar to the same enzyme in plants and mammals—is "sterol insensitive," that is, it does not switch off when there is an excess of steroid molecules. However, plants have learned that essential oil terpenes can switch this enzyme off. Plant terpenes are able to fight fungal attacks by shutting down their steroid synthesis, which thereby inhibits fungal growth.

When Elson and Peffley observed that the sterol insensitive HMG CoA reductase of tumor cells resembled that of fungi, they concluded that the reproduction of the tumor cells might be inhibited with essential oil components in much the same fashion as plants inhibit fungal reproduction. For an in-depth discussion of the ability of essential oils to modify the activity of HMG CoA reductase, and their effect on tumor growth in general, see Elson and Peffley in *Essential Oils and Cancer, Proceedings of the 4th Aromatherapy Conference on the Therapeutic Uses of Essential Oils*, 2000.[2]

The Work of Anne-Marie Giraud-Robert

The contention that essential oils are of great value to heal or treat cancer received an enormous boost through the work of French physician Dr. Anne-Marie Giraud-Robert, whose study was presented at the 7th Scientific Aromatherapy Conference on Essential Oils, Cancer, Degenerative, and Autoimmune Diseases, in 2009.[3] More than 1,800 cancer patients, who received allopathic treatment concurrently with essential oil treatment, had significantly higher survival rates than patients with comparative cancers and allopathic treatment alone. These observations were true for lung, colon, uterine, and breast cancer, as well as for all other types of cancer that were observed.

Dr. Giraud-Robert uses essential oils principally to reduce the often-debilitating side effects of conventional treatments. These side effects can be of such severity that they limit the use of the conventional medicines. It can be argued that reducing the side effects of the conventional

Pamela L. Crowell on the Prevention and Therapy of Cancer by Dietary Monoterpenes

Pamela L. Crowell of the biology department of Indian University is another leading researcher in the field of antitumor effects of mono- and sesquiterpene components. The following excerpt from one of her review papers is included to give the reader an idea how this research is communicated in its original form.[4]

Monoterpenes are non-nutritive dietary components found in the essential oils of citrus fruits and other plants. A number of these dietary monoterpenes have anti-tumor activity. For example, d-limonene, which comprises >90% of orange peel oil, has chemopreventive activity against rodent mammary, skin, liver, lung and forestomach cancers.

Similarly, other dietary monoterpenes have chemopreventive activity against rat mammary, lung, and forestomach cancers when fed during the initiation phase. In addition, perillyl alcohol has promotion phase chemopreventive activity against rat liver cancer, and geraniol has in vivo anti-tumor activity against murine leukemia cells. Perillyl alcohol and d-limonene also have chemotherapeutic activity against rodent mammary and pancreatic tumors. As a result, their cancer chemotherapeutic activities are under evaluation in Phase I clinical trials. Several mechanisms of action may account for the anti-tumor activities of monoterpenes. The blocking chemopreventive effects of limonene and other monoterpenes during the initiation phase of mammary carcinogenesis are likely due to the induction of Phase II carcinogen-metabolizing enzymes, resulting in carcinogen detoxification.

The post-initiation phase, tumor suppressive chemopreventive activity of monoterpenes may be due to the induction of apoptosis or to inhibition of the post-translational isoprenylation of cell growth-regulating proteins. Chemotherapy of chemically induced mammary tumors with monoterpenes results in tumor redifferentiation concomitant with increased expression of the mannose-6-phosphate/insulin-like growth factor II receptor and transforming growth factor ß1. Thus, monoterpenes would appear to act through multiple mechanisms in the chemoprevention and chemotherapy of cancer.

In summary, a variety of dietary monoterpenes have been shown to be effective in the chemoprevention and chemotherapy of cancer. Now, monoterpene research is progressing into human clinical trials for chemotherapeutic activity.

Monoterpenes also possess many characteristics of ideal chemopreventive agents, namely, efficacious anti-tumor activity, commercial availability, low cost, oral bioavailability and low toxicity, making it feasible to begin considering them for human cancer chemoprevention testing.

treatment allows patients to better tolerate those treatments, which ultimately leads to better outcomes.

Essential Oils in Cancer Treatment: When and Why

The issue of using essential oils to alleviate symptoms connected to cancer has been weighing heavily on the mind of many passionate aromatherapy users. The promise of benefits stands against the concern that one might cause more harm than good, as the essential oil components might produce undesirable drug interactions. These concerns have now been answered by Giraud-Robert's research results. Her studies show that patients who are treated with essential oils in addition to allopathic treatment have a dramatically improved prognosis.

Giraud-Robert suggests that aromatherapy should be viewed as a part of what she calls "backup care": "Backup care aims to ensure the best quality of life possible for patients in the physical, psychological, and social spheres every moment of their lives. In oncology, the treatment objective always has to be twofold, attempting to cure the disease and to maintain as high a life quality as possible."[5] Maintaining quality of life is difficult, as the conventional therapies attack not only the cancerous cells but also the healthy cells and drastic side effects are more the norm than the exception. Giraud-Robert's work is the first of its kind, clearly demonstrating that essential oil treatments are best suited to protect the patient's quality of life at the various stages of the disease.

The debilitating side effects of conventional cancer treatments include excessive sedation, anxiety, and severe restlessness. There can be very unpleasant sensations of muscular quivering or impaired or disordered muscle tone that results in clumsy, awkward, or difficult movement and lack of coordination. Very prominent side effects of chemotherapy can also be vomiting, nausea, increased susceptibility to infection, and blood and liver toxicity.

Giraud-Robert concludes that essential oil treatments improve quality of life not only by reducing the side effects of cancer drugs but equally importantly by stimulating the natural defenses and draining toxins from liver and kidneys. With essential oil treatments an increased efficacy of conventional treatments was often observed, possibly improving the patient's chances of survival. According to Giraud-Robert, aromatherapy can be beneficially used in all of the following stages of cancer:

Aromatherapy Innovation

The 7th Scientific Aromatherapy Conference on Essential Oils, Cancer, Degenerative, and Autoimmune Diseases in 2009 picked up where the abandoned research of the 1990s left off.

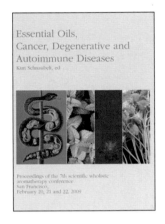

Pleiotropic Effects in Cancer Care

The pleiotropic nature of essential oils (see chapter 3) is of the utmost benefit in cancer care. Many aspects of the condition and the associated discomfort are ameliorated with one natural substance. Most essential oils have multiple beneficial effects, including acting against infectious organisms, thereby reducing the risk of secondary and opportunistic infection. They may help with sedation, pain relief, congestion, expectoration, tissue healing, and scar reduction, and they act as gentle antidepressants and help stimulate the appetite.

- Pre- or postoperative
- During and after chemotherapy
- During radiation therapy
- During immunotherapy treatment
- During hormonotherapy treatment
- During comfort care

The following suggestions in this chapter are those Dr. Giraud-Robert reported in her study.

Essential Oils for Cancer

Certain essential oils are particularly suited to be used alongside conventional cancer treatments, so they are described here.

Ravintsara (*Cinnamomum camphora*)

Ravintsara reduces physical and mental asthenia, which in turn helps the patient make decisions and regain self-confidence. During treatment, it counteracts depression. Ravintsara is sedating, promotes sleep, and improves sleep quality, and it reduces anxiety. Its antiviral activity and general improvement of immune response significantly reduce the risk of infection during chemotherapy. Ravintsara reduces most side effects of interferon treatment, such as depression, insomnia, muscle pains, and fatigue. It reduces joint pains and stiffness caused by antiaromatase-type antihormonal treatment for breast cancer. At the end of classical treatment, it stimulates the patient's immune system.

Greenland Moss (*Ledum groenlandicum*)

Greenland Moss is very effective for lessening nausea and vomiting during chemotherapy; it reduces pathologically elevated levels of transaminase and gamma-GT enzymes. It apparently acts as an antitumor agent by inducing cellular apoptosis. After conventional treatments, it is effective for draining the liver and kidneys.

Everlasting (*Helichrysum italicum*)

Helichrysum essential oil is extremely useful after surgery for reducing hematomas, improving healing, preventing cheloid scars, reducing lymphatic edemas following cleaning or dissecting of lymph nodes, and preventing fibrous bands in abdominal surgeries. Helichrysum is most useful in breast reconstruction, for its anti-inflammative, painkilling, and antiedematous effect and to eliminate old, hardened hematomas. Psychologically speaking, it soothes the soul's "bruises" and helps with emotional shocks.

Niaouli (*Melaleuca quinquenervia viridiflora*)

Massages with oils containing Niaouli reduce lymphatic edemas. Niaouli stimulates the immune response. It prevents radio epidermatitis during radiation therapy. It reduces the breast reconstruction period. Niaouli has powerful anti-infectious, antibacterial, antiviral, and antimycotic properties.

Myrrh (*Commiphora molmol*)

Myrrh is equally valuable during and after conventional treatment. It drains toxins from the kidneys during and after chemotherapy. Myrrh stimulates the nervous system and has antidepressant properties. It has strong analgesic properties. Myrrh has a very profound effect on a person's entire being by reequilibrating the psycho-neuro-endocrino-immunological systems. Myrrh induces cellular apoptosis.

Essential Oils and Chemotherapy

Chemotherapy protocols vary with the type of tumor, the stage of the disease, the patient's age, his or her general status, and visceral defects. The side effects of chemotherapy can be acute, arising during the first hours following chemotherapy. They can also be delayed, appearing after several chemotherapy cycles. They include digestive toxicity, blood cell toxicity, infections, neurotoxicity, and toxicity of the skin and nails.

Reducing Digestive Toxicity
Vomiting and Nausea

Chemotherapies generally induce nausea and vomiting, especially the anthracyclines and platinum salts. The nausea is generally reduced with allopathic drugs such as Zophren, Kytril, Emend, Solumedrol, and Vogalene. These treatments are even more effective when accompanied by an aromatherapy treatment. Dosage can be reduced and a corresponding reduction in side effects is observed.

Suggested Oils to Reduce Liver Toxicity

Essential oils of *Ledum groenlandicum* (Greenland Moss), *Citrus limon* (Lemon), *Rosmarinus officinalis* verbenone (Rosemary verbenone) are taken at a rate of 3 drops 3 times a day for 10 days following chemotherapy. Using these oils generally lowers the elevated levels of transaminase enzymes or gamma GT.

Suggested Oils for Ulcers or Canker Sores in the Oral Cavity

Essential oil preparations of Bay Laurel (*Laurus nobilis*), Carrot Seed (*Daucus carota*), Tea Tree (*Melaleuca alternifolia*), Niaouli (*Melaleuca quinquenervia viridiflora*), and Roman Chamomile (*Chamaemelum nobile*) diluted in wheat germ vegetable oil applied locally to the aphthas or gargling with calendula tincture are effective for preventing or soothing aphthas. These mouthwashes could also be used along with classic care, which is alkaline mouthwash with sodium bicarbonate at 1.4%.

Suggested Oils to Restore Taste and Regain Appetite

The essential oils of *Artemisia dracunculus* (Tarragon) and *Laurus nobilis* (Bay Laurel) help recover the normal taste of food.

Essential oils such as *Pimpinella anisum* (Anise), *Mentha x piperita* (Peppermint), and *Ocimum basilicum* (Basil) are used at a rate of 1 drop per day to stimulate appetite.

Liver Complications

Liver complications brought on by chemotherapy have been described frequently. The hepatotoxicity of different chemotherapy drugs is difficult to specify; however, nitrosyl-ureas induce enzymatic disruptions.

Inflammation of the Oral Mucous Membranes (Mucositis)

Mucositis is among chemotherapy's frequent side effects. Mucositis is a manifestation of either the direct toxicity of the agent used or of secondary immunodepression, making it easier for mycoses to develop. Mucositis can occur with most protocols but is more frequent with methotrexate, ellipticine, continuous 5 FU (Fluorouracil), and Periwinkle alkaloids. The condition is often confined to the oral cavity but can spread to the entire digestive tract.

Diarrhea and Constipation

Diarrhea is relatively frequent during chemotherapy. It is frequent with 5 FU (Fluorouracil), oxaliplatin (Eloxatine), and also with irinotecan (Campto). Constipation is frequent and its causes are various. It may be caused by the cancer itself (digestive and peritoneal localizations, hypocalcaemia), changes in lifestyle brought on by the disease (food, confinement to bed), and drugs such as opioids, chemotherapy, and related products.

In fact, antiemetics (substances effective against vomiting and nausea), especially setrons, can be responsible for constipative phenomena that are sometimes lasting and tenacious. Their role, as well as that of certain cytotoxics that slow bowel movements, must be determined, particularly that of Periwinkle alkaloids (vincristine, vinblastine, vindesine, vinorelbine). Constipation linked to cytotoxics is often accompanied by abdominal pains, nausea, and vomiting. The essential oil of *Ocimum basilicum* (Basil) helps keep bowel movements regular.

Appetite Loss and Altered Sense of Taste

Digestive problems can also impact appetite. In addition many drugs alter the sense of taste, such as doxetaxel (Taxotere).

Reducing Blood Cell Toxicity

Toxicity of the blood and blood forming tissues is most frequently chemotherapy's limiting factor. Blood toxicity is generally more pronounced in older patients, especially in the event of neoplastic (abnormal growth)

marrow infiltration or associated marrow pathology. The clinical indicator is an abnormally low count of specific white blood cells, especially neutrophils (neutropenia) or lymphocytes (lymphopenia), as well as a very low count of platelets (thrombopenia) or hemoglobin deficiency (anemia).

The point when the neutrophilic leukocyte count reaches its lowest point is called the nadir. It is generally observed eight to ten days after chemotherapy. The duration and severity of this neutropenia depends on the type of chemotherapy drug used as well as its dosage. Associated with neutropenia is the risk of infection-related complications.

Thrombopenia is generally offset by a few days from the neutropenia. The risk of bleeding is especially pronounced when the platelet count drops below 20,000 platelets per cubic millimeter.

Anemia induced by chemotherapy comes in addition to anemia associated with cancer: anemia caused by chronic digestive deficiency.

Prevention of Infections and Their Complications

Complications originating from infections remain an everyday problem in oncology. The causes of these infections are many: the cancer lesions themselves (for example, bronchial tumors, ORL tumors), reduction in immune defenses associated with the underlying pathology or with nonspecific problems such as malnutrition, invasive diagnostic or therapeutic activity, or implementations such as central catheters. Neutropenias following chemotherapy also promote infections.

Reducing Neurotoxicity

Toxicity affecting the nervous system can be observed in the central, the peripheral, and the autonomic nervous system. Symptoms affecting the higher brain functions may be observed with ifosfamide (Holoxan) and assume the form of confusion or delirium.

Symptoms in the peripheral nervous system (the nerves and ganglia outside of the brain and spinal cord, which connect the central nervous system to the limbs and organs) are observed with Periwinkle alkaloids: vincristine, vindesine, vinblastine, and, to a lesser degree, vinorelbine, paclitaxel, cisplatin, and oxaliplatin. The latter triggers peripheral and vegetative symptoms (symptoms caused by imbalances of the autonomic nervous system) under the influence of cold: that is, prickling or tingling (paresthesia) when the hands reach into the refrigerator. This may also take the form of laryngeal spasm while drinking cold drinks. These symptoms,

Suggested Oils to Reduce Hematologic Toxicity

Essential Oils of *Cinnamomum camphora* (Ravintsara) and *Commiphora molmol* (Myrrh) reduce hematologic toxicity, 3 drops twice a day for the 10 days following chemotherapy.

Suggested Oils to Prevent Infections

Essential oils such as the essential oil of *Cinnamomum camphora* (Ravintsara) and the essential oil of *Thymus vulgaris* type thujanol (Thyme thujanol) and the essential oil of *Cymbopogon martinii* (Palmarosa) are taken, 2 drops each twice a day for the 10 days following chemotherapy. They are useful for preventing infections.

Suggested Oils for Polyneuritis

Polyneuritis (the inflammation of multiple nerves, marked by paralysis, pain, and muscle wasting) is very difficult to alleviate. Results have sometimes been obtained using the following essential oils: *Cryptomeria japonica* (Japanese cedar), *Ferula galbaniflua* (Galbanum), and *Helichrysum italicum* (Everlasting) diluted in vegetable oil and used with massage.

which often start with paresthesia of the extremities, can, particularly with cisplatin, become serious (superficial or deep) and irreversible impairments of the motor and sensory apparatus. Other vegetative symptoms such as constipation or laryngeal spasm have already been mentioned.

Reducing Toxicity of the Skin and Nails

Chemotherapy drugs that cause skin and nail problems mostly are the taxanes, especially docetaxel (Taxotere) as well as cepecitabine (Xeloda), and 5 FU.

Nail Problems

The drugs mentioned cause brown hyperpigmentation, malformation of nails, separation of the nail from its bed, and pain in the extremities.

Skin Problems of the Hands and Feet

Certain chemotherapies and targeted therapies (which block the growth and spread of cancer by interfering with specific molecules involved in tumor growth and progression) cause trophic skin disorders of the extremities such as hand-foot syndrome (also called palmar plantar erythrodysesthesia). This syndrome was described for the first time in 1974. In most cases (about 80 percent), hand-foot syndrome is low grade (Grade 1 according to the National Cancer Institute's criteria).

TOXICITY CLASSIFICATION OF HAND-FOOT SYNDROME (NCI)

Grade 1
Mild erythema, swelling, or desquamation that does not interfere with daily activities.

Grade 2
Erythema, desquamation, or swelling that interferes with, but does not prevent, normal physical activities: small blisters or ulcerations of less than three quarters of an inch in diameter.

Grade 3
Blister, ulceration, or swelling that interferes with walking or normal daily activities; cannot wear usual clothes.

Grade 4
Diffuse or local, leading to complications with confinement to bed or hospitalization.

Palmar plantar syndrome can be deleterious in terms of quality of life during chemotherapy. The chemotherapy drugs mostly responsible for the hand-foot syndrome are cepecitabine (Xeloda), topotecan (Hycamtin), docetaxel (Taxotere), and paclitaxel (Taxol). Targeted therapies such as cetuximab (Erbitux), erlotinib (Tarceva), sorafenib (Nexavar), and sunitinib (Sutent) are also responsible for the hand-foot syndrome.

Drug-Induced Acne

The use of anti-VEGF monoclonal (single species) antibodies, or anti-EGF, has caused new side effects: purulent acne of the face and upper part of the body. This side effect, which is seen as a sign of the effectiveness of the treatment, can be treated with aromatherapy, thereby avoiding a prescription of doxycycline. The main molecules used in chemotherapy that give rise to acne are azathioprine (Imurel), cepecitabine (Xeloda), and methotrexate (Ledertrexate, Metoject, Novatrex). Among the monoclonal antibodies, bevacizumab (Avastin), cetuximab (Erbitux), erlotinib (Tarceva), and trastuzumab (Herceptin) cause the most acne.

Skin and Lip Dryness and Cracks

5 FU (Fluoro-uracil) and irinotecan (Campto) (FOLFIRI protocol) used in cancers of the colon cause skin dryness with "face powder" desquamation (the skin peeling off in powdery scales). Treatments using a strong dose of methotrexate and using anti-EGFR monoclonal antibodies also cause skin dryness, blotches on the face, and cracks on the lips.

Edemas

Edemas and effusions of the serous membranes (membranes covering the internal cavities of the body) linked to docetaxel (Taxotere) that appear cumulatively are successfully prevented or slowed by systematic oral corticoid therapy surrounding the cytotoxic's drip. In the event of a pleural or peritoneal seeping of fluid, the cytology will perform the differential diagnosis between effusion linked to docetaxel (Taxotere) or neoplastic localization. These edemas and effusions generally only recede when the docetaxel is stopped.

Suggested Oils for Acne

Application of Lavender hydrosol is very useful on the acne area. For local application on each acne pimple: *Melaleuca alternifolia* (Tea Tree), *Daucus carota* (Carrot), *Helichrysum italicum* (Everlasting), and *Melaleuca quinquenervia viridiflora* (Niaouli).

Suggested Oils for Dryness and Cracks

Jojoba oil hydrates the skin well. For cracks and plantar keratosis (horny growths at the sole of the foot), essential oils of Cypress (*Cupressus sempervirens*), Tea Tree (*Melaleuca alternifolia*), and Everlasting (*Helichrysum italicum*), diluted in vegetable oil, speed up healing of the cracks.

Suggested Oils for Edema

Take the following essential oils orally or massage with the oils diluted in vegetable oil to reduce edemas linked to docetaxel: *Citrus limon* (Lemon), *Helichrysum italicum* (Everlasting), *Melaleuca alternifolia* (Tea Tree), *Melaleuca quinquenervia viridiflora* (Niaouli).

Suggested Oils for Nosebleed

Essential oil of Rock Rose (*Cistus ladaniferus*), 2 to 3 drops on a cotton wick, will stop epistaxis.

Suggested Oils for Alopecia

Massaging the scalp with essential oils of *Melaleuca quinquenervia viridiflora* (Niaouli), *Melaleuca alternifolia* (Tea Tree), and *Helichrysum italicum* (Everlasting) diluted 10% in vegetable oil reduces the unpleasant sensations associated with hair loss.

Niaouli Essential Oil for Radiation Therapy

Essential oil of Niaouli (*Melaleuca quinquenervia viridiflora*) is very effective for reducing certain side effects of radiation therapy, especially those that appear during irradiation.

Suggested Oils for Wounds and Burns

For wounds or burns, the essential oils of *Pogostemon cablin* (Patchouli), *Cistus ladaniferus* (Rock Rose), and *Lavandula spica* (Spike Lavender) are very effective (pure or diluted).

Epistaxis (Nose Bleed)

Some treatments cause epistaxis, like bevacizumab (Avastatin).

Drug-Induced Alopecia (Hair Loss)

Chemotherapy-induced alopecia can be total, but is generally reversible. The regrowth can be accompanied by a change in the texture and color of the hair. It can spread to body hair, eyelashes, and eyebrows during treatment using taxanes. If the hair loss cannot be stopped by aromatherapy, the latter can bring some relief to certain unpleasant symptoms, particularly during the time when the hair falls out and when it grows back. The scalp is often hypersensitive when the hair falls out and grows back, which can lead to pain.

Radiation Therapy

While radiation is decreasingly being used as a sole treatment, more than 70 percent of patients treated for a malignant tumor will undergo radiation therapy once or several times during the course of their illness. This may be at the initial stage along with surgery or with chemotherapy. Radiation is also very frequently used during a metastatic phase for treating bone or brain metastases.

Traditionally, the distinction is made between acute effects, which appear during irradiation, and delayed effects, which appear afterward. Acute effects depend on the irradiated organs and appear during irradiation and normally disappear without aftereffects in the weeks following the irradiation.

Acute Effects of Radiation

The acute effects of radiation include damage to the skin, appearance of an edema, mucositis, or esophagitis, or digestive disturbance, depending on the location of the radiation.

Skin damage caused by irradiation is well known. Initially a simple erythema, similar to sunburn, is observed. A severe desquamation can occur.

Brain irradiation has the inherent risk of being followed by the appearance of an edema, which could lead to high blood pressure in the brain. Thorax irradiation is performed for esophageal or bronchopulmonary cancers. It rarely causes skin complications. The immediate response to this irradiation is often esophagitis, which also can be the cause of severe difficulty in swallowing (dysphagia), requiring artificial alimentation. Abdominal irradiation is frequently accompanied by nausea, vomiting, and diarrhea.

ORL (Otolaryngology) Radiation Therapy

Radiation-induced mucositis is initially represented by areas of severe redness (erythema), then ulcerations of the mucous membranes, which are isolated then confluent. Mucositis can cause pain, which may require major class II analgesics or even opioids, and difficulty in swallowing, which can justify tubal or intraveneous feeding. Microbial, candida, or herpes superinfection tends to occur along with mucositis and should ideally be prevented.

Irradiation of Breasts

Breast irradiation is normally accompanied by a skin inflammation or irritation (epithelitis), which can be anything from a simple redness to scaling. A mammary edema, more or less painful, is frequent. Fungal superinfection can occur in the mammary groove, if breasts are large or in older women.

UNDERSTANDING AROMATHERAPY

Other Oils for Breast Radiation Therapy

When Niaouli oil has not been applied from the beginning or when cutaneous lesions appear during radiation therapy in spite of applying it, applications of Everlasting hydrosol and Lavender hydrosol relieve the pain very quickly and improve the lesions within a few days. Applying essential oil of *Pogostemon cablin* (Patchouli), *Cistus ladaniferus* (Rock Rose), and *Lavandula spica* (Spike Lavender) diluted in a vegetable oil speeds up healing.

Pelvic Irradiation

Depending on the size of the irradiated area, pelvic irradiation can lead to nausea, vomiting, and diarrhea because of the presence of the small intestine in the pelvis minor. It can be the cause of radiation-induced cystitis with urinary burns and frequent urination (pollakiuria). Radiation-induced inflammation of the rectum (proctitis) is usually seen when this treatment is used for rectal cancer, gynecologic, or prostatic tumors. Pelvic irradiation results in local pains, an increase in the frequency of stools that are often liquid, and emission of phlegm. As a result of irradiation of the area between the anus and the genital organs (perineum), (to treat cancer of the anal canal, the lower rectum, the vulva, or vagina), perineal inflammation is sometimes severe.

Delayed Effects of Irradiation

The delayed effects of radiation can include skin, breast, ORL, dental, thoracic, and digestive complications and metastatic cancers. Radiation-induced epithelitis usually disappears in two or three weeks. It can, however, be followed by a permanent, often mild, cutaneous pigmentation. Bluish red spots (telangiectasias) can appear several years after irradiation has been stopped.

Dryness of the mouth (xerostomia) is the rule after irradiation for ORL or stomatological cancer. Dental problems are not rare after irradiation; they should be prevented by applying fluorine gel.

Radiation-induced respiratory disease (pneumopathy) usually arises two or three months after irradiation has been stopped. Clinically, coughing and intermittent fever (febricula) are the principal symptoms, but an exertional shortness of breath (dyspnea) sometimes appears along with them. Radiation-induced esophagitis can be complicated by a narrowing of the esophagus with the formation of excessive fibrous tissue (fibrotic stenosis), which can require repeated widening.

Digestive problems such as diarrhea or abdominal pains can occur after irradiation. Radiation-induced inflammation of the rectum and anus is seen mainly after prostate cancer irradiation: it manifests most often as episodic discharge, occurring two to three times a week.

Metastatic Cancers

Metastatic cancers are rare and are seen mainly after irradiation of Hodgkin's disease. They occur ten to twenty-five years after treatment. Giraud-Robert, however, points out the very great risk of breast cancer for young women irradiated on the chest before the age of twenty, which justifies a regular and careful examination of these patients' breasts.

Essential Oils and Interferon

Interferon treatment is often prescribed to treat certain stages of melanoma. The undesirable effects of interferon are often significant, sometimes making it necessary to reduce the dosage, which in turn could reduce the treatment's effectiveness. The most frequently encountered side effects are:

- Pseudo-influenza syndrome (often increased at the beginning of treatment)
- Change in general status (reduced appetite, weight loss, asthenia)
- Significant neuropsychiatric symptoms

Neuropsychiatric symptoms include anxiety and depression. Often the status of the patient fluctuates unpredictably, independent of psychiatric history. Interferon leads to a lack of dopamine and serotonin. Other interferon side effects include sleep disorders, psychomotor agitation, problems with concentration and memory, aggressiveness, anxious asthenia with the inability to relax, and hypersomnia.

Specific Symptoms

The specific symptoms of interferon include fatigue, bone and joint pain, neuropathic, neurologic, and visceral pain, diffuse pain, and pseudo-influenzal syndromes. Fatigue is in most cases the main symptom of which patients complain. Its severity is often not fully recognized. Bone pain in a cancer patient can always be a sign of metastasis. But in most cases the injection of granulocyte growth factors like filgrastim (Neupogen) and especially its time release version, pegfilgrastim (Neulasta), cause bone pain, often of the wrenching type.

Thirty percent of patients undergoing anti-aromatase adjuvant hormonotherapy experience joint and tendon/muscle pains. These drugs, such as anastrozole (Arimidex) or letrozole (Femara), which block the enzyme aromatase that produces estrogen, are generally prescribed for menopausal breast cancer patients. These pains are sometimes very significant, necessitating a change of treatment.

The appearance of shingles is a frequent consequence of chemotherapy-induced immunodepression, and patients often suffer from incapacitating post-zoster pains.

UNDERSTANDING AROMATHERAPY

Essential Oils for Interferon Side Effects

Essential oils such as *Ledum groenlandicum* (Greenland Moss) and *Cinnamomum camphora* (Ravintsara) help reduce interferon's side effects.

UNDERSTANDING AROMATHERAPY

Essential Oils for Fatigue

Essential oils of Greenland Moss, Ravintsara, and Peppermint are useful for reducing fatigue.

Prescribing chemotherapy by mouth is very convenient for the patient, but is sometimes accompanied by digestive disorders and abdominal pains. Abdominal metastases, in particular peritoneal ones, are also very painful.

We have seen that, in the hours following injection, immunomodulator treatments, cytokines like interferon alpha, cause a pseudo-influenzal syndrome with myalgia, fever, and asthenia.

Essential Oils for Comfort Care

Often comfort care is considered synonymous with end-of-life treatments. But comfort care includes all situations where a corrective solution does not exist, including patients who have tumors along with a very long life expectancy. After allopathic treatments have ended, it is also always important to drain the organism and work on the patient's immune system.

For the WHO (World Health Organization), comfort care consists of active care for those patients whose illness is not responding to a corrective or curative treatment. In those scenarios the management of pain is essential, and psychosocial and spiritual issues need to be given proper attention with the goal of allowing a better quality of life for the patients as well as their families.

In the experience of many workgroups it has been learned that the quality of life assessment must be centered on the patient and his or her family. Support for a person at the end-of-life stage and for his or her family and friends consists of paying attention, listening, and comforting, while taking into account the components of the overall suffering. These will often be pain phenomena. Sometimes bouts of hiccups can be relieved by using the oils of Melissa or *Artemisia dracunculus*. It is very important to take care of the patient during this period because it is often the period when the patient can feel abandoned. Studies in Great Britain, in palliative care facilities, have shown that aromatherapy massage with the essential oil of *Lavandula vera* (Lavender absolute) improved quality of life and reduced psychological distress.

FOURTEEN

SELECTED ASPECTS OF CHINESE MEDICAL AROMATHERAPY

Cancer and Autoimmune Diseases

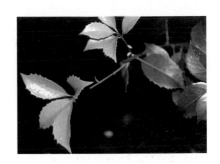

Tea is the most popular beverage, after water, throughout the world. Not surprisingly, there is a rich mythology surrounding the history of tea and its important role in many cultures of the world.

LESTER A. MITSCHER AND VICTORIA DOLBY

Unlike other healing systems, which are built around a single concept, Chinese medicine, due to its historical development, entertains various models of recognition and action. There are anatomical models focusing on concepts such as inside to outside, extremities to trunk, or skin to marrow. Another model focuses on organs (Zang-Fu) and yet another one on the humors: qi, blood, body fluids, *jing* (essence), and *shen* (spirit). Jing (essence) and shen (spirit) are terms that describe elements and processes transcending the physical. For more expansive narratives on these subjects, please consult the ample literature on Chinese medicine.

Chinese Medicine and Cancer

When it comes to cancer, the viewpoint of Chinese medicine is instructive. To avoid lengthy dissertations, only some central considerations are presented. Readers who find them too esoteric are encouraged to either ignore them or, if interested, to satisfy their curiosity by digging into the phenomenal depths of this healing system.

Fuzheng therapy strengthens immunity, clears tumors (called fire toxins), and promotes elimination. Treatments revolve around supporting (*fu*) the upright (*zheng*) qi. If the patient is too weak to tolerate full resolution of the disease the aim is to keep the pathogenic processes latent, preventing a worsening of the status. Full resolution of the disease by stimulating the elimination of accumulated pathogens (fire toxins) should only be attempted for patients with adequate upright qi. Essential oils suggested by Jeffrey Yuen to clear fire toxins are Celery Seed, *Helichrysum italicum,* Lovage, Mimosa, Palmarosa, Sage, Atlas Cedar, Bay Laurel, Elemi, *Eucalyptus polybractea,* Grapefruit, and Orange. Yuen also reiterates that these oils do not represent treatment per se for cancerous processes but can only be seen within the context of traditional Chinese medicine (TCM), which addresses each patient individually.

In the Taoist approach the person is treated, not the disease. Looking at the patient first often leads to the realization that she or he is too weak to attempt resolution of the cancer itself. Treating the cancer would kill the patient, an occurrence all too familiar in Western medicine. Treating the patient instead of the cancer may indicate the need to embrace latency, that is, not to try to eliminate the cancer immediately, but instead to maintain the status quo while strengthening the patient. Only at a later point, when the patient has been returned to a state of sufficient strength, is the treatment or elimination of the cancer attempted.

To better understand the relation of essential oils to the tumor phenomenon from the viewpoint of Chinese medicine, it is helpful to recognize that the Taoist cultivator considers the essence of the plant to be a representation of its yuan qi (its original qi) or, in Western terms, of its genetic code. Within this formalism the essence of the plant is seen to "resonate" with the yuan qi of humans, helping to maintain the integrity of the yuan qi. Combining the results of Elson and Peffley—indicating that the reproduction of tumor cells might be inhibited with essential oil components, similar to the way plants inhibit fungal reproduction—with the insight of Chinese medicine produces one immediately applicable conclusion: using essential oils on a daily basis appears to be one of the most useful measures to prevent cancer.

From a purely mechanistic perspective, essential oils with high concentrations of limonene, such as Lemon or Orange, should be considered. But, again, the research links the highest efficacy to the dietary intake of a diverse mixture of terpenoids!

Autoimmune Conditions: A Chinese Medical Perspective

This presentation of a classical Chinese medical view of addressing autoimmune diseases is adapted from a presentation on Chinese medical aromatherapy, given by Jeffrey Yuen in San Francisco in 2006.

Western medicine recognizes many different autoimmune conditions like lupus or Crohn's disease. It logs symptoms and suggests treatments specific to the condition. Chinese medicine recognizes the common thread of these conditions: our body prevents pathogens from entering the inner organs by making them dormant in the external parts of the body, where they are not necessarily as dangerous. We become aware of this when the body makes occasional attempts to eliminate the pathogen (flare-up). However, it never fully gets rid of it.

Areas where autoimmune conditions typically manifest are skin (scleroderma), muscles (muscular dystrophy), joints (arthritis), or the mucous membranes (colitis). These conditions are marked by intermittent flare-ups and asymptomatic periods. During flare-ups patients often feel lethargic. Resting leads to improved well-being. Once the body has gained new strength, it often responds with a new, but generally unsuccessful, attempt to eliminate the pathogen.

Flare-ups are brought on by the release of histamine, which stimulates discharge and inflammation. The general response of Western medicine is to resort to steroid drugs (cortisone), which inhibit histamine release and thereby suppress discharge, simultaneously increasing tolerance to the pathogen. Steroid drugs lead to autointoxication.

The Chinese medical approach acknowledges the body's aggressive reactions, which are nonetheless insufficient for the complete elimination of the pathogen. As a first response, Chinese medicine attempts to modulate (not inhibit) the histamine release so that the patient should not have to resort to steroid drugs. This is done by redirecting, "grounding," the body's defensive energy (wei qi), which can be influenced via the area in proximity to the lumbar spine.

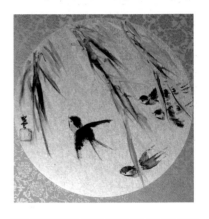
Selected Aspects of Chinese Medical Aromatherapy

Ubiquitous Rose

Plant life radiates into all directions where the seeds find viable environments to germinate. Similarly the myths connected to plants of foreign lands are often eagerly soaked up in locales halfway around the planet. Below is a California stained glass piece inspired by the innumerable myths about the Rose (original glass art by Monika Haas).

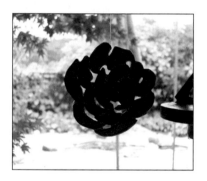

Containing Excessive Wei Qi

Anchoring a hypervigilant immune system is the first step in the treatment of autoimmune conditions. Oils are applied to the base of the spine, especially to the right and left of the lower spine. Massaging with root oils such as Spikenard and Vetiver in a downward motion along the lumbar spine moves defensive energy downward and contains excessive immune response. Drawing energy down and inward reduces outward directed defensive energy (wei qi), ameliorating the hypervigilance of the immune system. Astringent essential oils such as Cistus, Cypress, or Benzoin help to draw energy inward. Treatment with these essential oils often breaks open stagnant states of the mind, exposing the core issues underlying the condition!

At this stage it is also important to adhere to a diet that does not stimulate defensive energy; it should be free of highly stimulant spices, such as garlic.

The Pathogenic Factor

A pathogenic factor in this Chinese view can be many things: a microorganism or environmental toxin, and also stress. Identifying the nature of the pathogen is essential for its ultimate elimination. In industrial urban societies stress factors are often at the core of the original problem. The body of the patient has been overwhelmed and confused for long periods of time, continuously remaining active, not knowing how to slow down. "How can I do all of this?" is a desperate sigh of such individuals. Ultimately permanent stresses cause physical and mental exhaustion, chronic stress syndrome, or autoimmune taxation. This causality is also increasingly recognized in Western medicine and termed repetitive stress injury (RSI).

Continuation of the Treatment

The next step is to strengthen the patient to make successful elimination of the pathogen feasible. To expel the pathogen the body needs sufficient fluid resources, sufficient blood, hormones, and exocrine fluids. It is necessary to strengthen these resources or, in the language of Chinese medicine, to increase the body's substantiations.

This may involve building blood and stimulating the hormone system as well as hydrating the body to support secretions of the so-called thin fluids, that is urine, saliva, sweat, and fluids secreted through eyes

Western Classification of Autoimmune Conditions

Fundamentally different from Chinese medicine, the Western view does not include a unifying concept to explain autoimmune diseases but instead lists many categories of such conditions, generally based on their different symptoms.

Organ-Specific Autoimmune Diseases

Endocrine Glands:

Hashimoto's Thyroiditis

Basedow Syndrome

Addison's Disease

Insulin-dependent Diabetes

Skin:

Pemphigus

Pemphigoid

Vitiligo

Hematopoietic Organs (spleen, lymph nodes, etc.):

Hemolytic Anemia

Leukopenia

Thrombopenia

Central Nervous System:

Multiple Sclerosis

Myastenia

Digestive Tract and Liver:

Biermer's Anemia

Chronic Autoimmune Hepatitis

Billiary Cirrhosis

Crohn's Disease

Hemorrhagic Rectocolitis

Non Organ-Specific Autoimmune Diseases

Systemic Lupus

Gougerot-Sjögren Syndrome

Rheumatoid Polyarthritis

Horton's Disease and Rhizomelic Pseudo-Polyarthritis

Scleroderma

Weakening Polymysotis

Selected Aspects of Chinese
Medical Aromatherapy

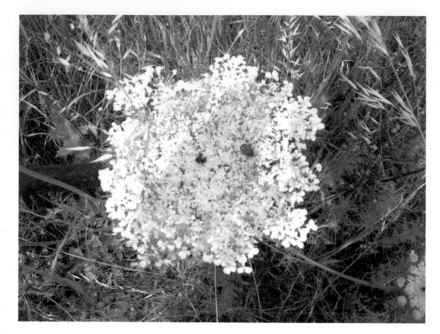

Building blood: Essential oil of Carrot Seed is recommended by Jeffrey Yuen to increase the body's substantiations. (The white flowers of the carrot plant feature a black spot in the middle, which apparently tricks passing bugs into stopping!)

and nose (exocrine fluids). Savory and Carrot Seed are essential oils used to build blood, and *Vitex agnus castus* can be employed to balance and strengthen the endocrine (hormonal) system. Geranium can be used to nurture fluid levels.

Only when there is enough moisture, proper hormonal balance, and sufficient blood should a flushing out of the pathogenic factor be initiated. If the body is not sufficiently hydrated to support flushing, the healing crisis will be too strong and the patient will likely revert back to the vicious cycle of steroids and flare-ups. To determine whether the body is sufficiently hydrated, the presentation of lips and mouth (dry or moist), bronchi (dry or moist), and eyes and nose along with their associated mucous membranes is considered.

Once the determination has been made to attempt elimination of the pathogenic factor, essential oils can be used to trigger wei qi. Depending on the condition, different essential oils may be appropriate:

- For metabolic conditions and to help elimination from liver and digestive tract: Rosemary verbenone
- To draw chronically lodged viruses from tissue or to draw a pathogenic factor from bones: Clove
- To draw biological pathogens or lactic acid from muscles and joints: *Litsea cubeba,* Lemon verbena, or Spruce

- To draw inorganic toxins such as uric acids and mineral-type deposits: Celery Seed (or Celery juice can also be effective)
- For conditions manifesting on the skin: camphor or oils with a pronounced camphor character, such as *Lavandula spica* or *Lavandula stoechas*

Discharge of the Pathogenic Factor

In the view of Chinese medicine any number of discharge processes, involving exocrine fluid or also blood, can participate in the elimination of the pathogenic factor, depending on the specific condition and the patient.

It may need to be noted that in Chinese medicine there appears to be a broader acceptance of the sometimes rather cathartic discharge processes than in the Western view. Discharge processes involving blood may involve strong and very strong menstruation, but also loss of blood through nose bleeds or rectal bleeding (especially in the case of preexisting hemorrhoids). Discharge involving exocrine fluids may involve urine, sweating, elimination of fluid or mucus from lungs, nose, or eyes, but also diarrhea and vomiting.

Summing Up

When overwhelming stress depletes the blood, endocrine, and exocrine fluid resources of our body to the point that they become inadequate to support the complete elimination of a pathogenic factor, autoimmune disease is the result. Without the chance to fully eliminate the pathogenic factor, our immune system periodically attempts to resolve the condition. Considering that the pathogenic factor had taken up residency over long periods of time and created its own manifestations in the life of a human body, it is not too surprising that the elimination processes that are necessary to truly get rid of it sometimes take on dramatic forms.

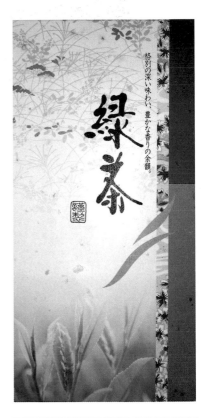

PLANTS IN ARTS AND CULTURE

Camellia sinensis

The many representations in cultures around the globe of plant imagery are testimony to the intense interaction between plant and human life. It has been argued that the course of development of Buddhism cannot be imagined absent its close connection to the *Camellia sinensis* plant.

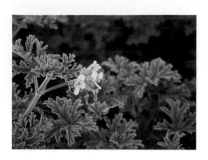

FIFTEEN

ESSENTIAL OILS AND HEPATITIS B AND C

Simply put, their spirit is manifest in their authenticity.

ANTHONY F. GRANUCCI,

THE ART OF THE LESSER SUNDAS

As we have seen, essential oils interact with many processes in the liver. Their induction and inhibition of Phase I and II detoxification enzymes is but one example. Traditional knowledge asserts that certain oils, most importantly Carrot Seed and Greenland Moss, do in some way support the regeneration of the liver. *L'aromathérapie exactement* also reports that Thyme thuyanol specifically stimulates liver regeneration. As the activity of essential oils with respect to liver health is clearly of the highest importance, a presentation Dr. Giraud-Robert gave at the International Symposium of Aromatherapy and Medicinal Plants, Grasse, in March 2005 is summarized here.[1]

Current Understanding of Hepatitis B and C

The viruses responsible for chronic hepatitis are called hepatitis B, C, D, and G virus. Hepatitis is considered chronic when transaminase counts are elevated above twice their normal ranges for more than six months. Hepatitis B and especially C represent an increasing problem in Western societies. Of individuals with hepatitis C, 85 to 90 percent go on to develop chronic hepatitis, whereas for hepatitis B the number is 5 to 10 percent for immunocompetent carriers. For hepatitis C, the current allopathic treatment is therapy with interferon and ribavirin. This leads to eradication of the virus in almost 85 percent of patients infected with genotype 2 or 3 and only 50 percent eradication in those with genotype 1. Negative side effects of these treatments are common. For hepatitis B, allopathic treatments rely on interferon and nucleoside analogues such as lamivudine and adefovir. The objective of treatment is to render the virus noninfective rather than virus eradication.

The study that Dr. Giraud-Robert presented at the symposium reported on 60 patients who were chronic carriers of hepatitis B (10) or C (50). Essential oils such as Ravintsara, Greenland Moss, Carrot Seed, and Thyme thuyanol were used as a complement to allopathic treatment. In patients with hepatitis C treated with interferon and essential oils, tolerance and response to treatment was improved (80 percent good tolerance and 100 percent complete response, especially for genotype 1). For hepatitis C patients who were only treated with essential oils, a significant improvement was noted in 64 percent of the cases. For hepatitis B, two cures were obtained with essential oil treatment only.

Dr. Giraud-Robert concluded that essential oils may offer therapeutic opportunities either as stand-alone therapy or as complement to allopathic interventions.

Hepatitis C

Hepatitis C is a relatively frequent infection. The hepatitis C virus is an RNA virus with a highly variable genome. This variability is the cause of the emergence of several genotypes, numbered 1 through 6. Transmission of hepatitis C is essentially through the blood. The two main modes of transmission are intravenous drug use and contaminated blood transfusions. Transmission from mother to child is rare.

Hepatitis C is a disease whose evolution is extremely variable from one person to another and is often slow to progress. Infection with hepatitis C leads to inflammation of hepatocytes (cells of the liver lining). This may be acute or prolonged. The acute phase is usually asymptomatic.

Progression to a chronic state occurs in 85 to 90 percent of cases. This high rate of progression is due to the above-mentioned high genome variability. It is responsible for permanent mutations that permit this

RNA virus to escape immune defenses. In the absence of healing, the virus remains in the hepatocytes and the immune response provokes the typical lesions of chronic hepatitis. This chronic inflammation is responsible for a progressive fibrosis with scar tissue, which can end in cirrhosis of the liver that may remain undetected for years. Once cirrhosis is established, the incidence of developing hepatocellular carcinoma is 3 to 5 percent.

The conventional treatment as of 2005 consisted of associating interferon and ribavirin treatment. Success depended largely on the genotype of the virus. The actual viral load was also an important factor determining treatment success. Smaller viral load generally meant better response to treatment. Despite progress in recent years, the conventional treatments bring numerous, significant, usually dose-dependent negative side effects. The most common ones are listed in the table below.

SIDE EFFECTS OF CONVENTIONAL THERAPY

Side Effects Linked to Interferon	Side Effects Linked to Ribavirin
Pseudo-flu syndrome	Hemolytic anemia
Mood alteration and depression	Pruritis
Hypo- and hyperthyroidism	Teratogenicity
Other autoimmune disorders	Mitochondrial toxicity
Alopecia (partial)	
Anemia, leucopenia, thrombopenia	

Hepatitis B

Hepatitis B is a principal worldwide public health issue; approximately 350 million people are chronic carriers of hepatitis B. The hepatitis B virus is an enveloped DNA virus. Infection may occur by sexual, intravenous, or perinatal transmission.

Hepatitis B is a potentially serious disease due to its progression to chronic hepatitis; 5 to 10 percent of cases have the risk of evolution to cirrhosis or hepatic carcinoma. The initial infection is most often asymptomatic, but it may evolve to fulminant hepatitis that is usually fatal.

Essential Oils Included in the Study

The objective of Dr. Giraud-Robert's study was to demonstrate antiviral and antifibrotic activity of a number of essential oils when used either as a stand-alone therapy or alongside allopathic treatment for hepatitis.

The essential oils most often prescribed included Ravintsara, Greenland Moss, Thyme thuyanol, Bay Laurel, Carrot, Niaouli, and Helichrysum. They were taken orally, diluted in honey or vegetable oil, or in gel capsules. The dosage varied depending on the therapeutic properties of the different oils. Massage was used rarely, only if there was intolerance to the oral route.

Ravintsara was prescribed at 5 drops, 3 times per day, Bay Laurel at 1 drop per day, and Greenland Moss 3 drops, 3 times per day. Generally, Ravintsara and Greenland Moss were given together, representing the main thrust of the essential oil treatment, along with a third oil that was changed every three or four months. The essential oils were generally taken for one week every month. Giraud-Robert calls this week the "therapeutic window."

Following is a listing of the claimed or demonstrated properties that make these oils useful in the treatment of hepatitis.

Carrot (*Daucus carota*)

Claimed properties include: hepatocellular regeneration, general tonic, and stimulant. It lowers high cholesterol.

Traditional indications are for hepatic and renal insufficiency and skin disorders like burns and furuncles.

Bay Laurel (*Laurus nobilis*)

Claimed properties include: antibacterial, antiviral, fungicidal, analgesic, antineuralgic, mucolytic, and expectorant.

Traditional indications include: ear, nose, and throat infections, influenza, viral hepatitis, fungal infections of the skin, gynecological and digestive tract conditions.

Helichrysum (*Helichrysum italicum*)

Claimed properties include: antiedema, antispasmodic, and hepato-pancreatic stimulant.

Traditional indications include: hematomas, phlebitis, hepatocyte insufficiency, hepatitis, cirrhosis.

Niaouli (*Melaleuca quinquenervia viridiflora*)

Claimed properties include: antibacterial, antiviral, antifungal, radio-protectant and venous decongestant.

Traditional indications include: gynecological, cutaneous, and respiratory infections, viral hepatitis and radiodermatitis.

Thyme thuyanol (*Thymus vulgaris*)

Claimed properties include: antibacterial, antiviral, immune stimulant, hepatocyte tonic and regenerator, neurotonic.

Traditional indications include: gynecological, cutaneous, and respiratory infections, viral hepatitis and cirrhosis.

Indications for Stand-Alone Aromatherapy Treatment

Giraud-Robert considers stand-alone essential oil treatment appropriate in the following circumstances:

- Patients presenting with a definitive or temporary contraindication to conventional treatment
- Carriers of minimal hepatitis C (Metavir score of F0, F1, A0, A1) with no extra hepatic signs and if the person is not asking for treatment with interferon
- Carriers of minimal hepatitis B (healthy carriers, with normal transaminase counts) or patients refusing allopathic treatment in writing when it would normally be indicated for their status

Objectives of Essential Oil Treatments

The results of Dr. Giraud-Robert's work show that essential oil treatments in fact do reduce the transaminase count as well as the viral load. A second objective is the stabilization or regression of fibrosis.

In circumstances where essential oils were used in conjunction with conventional treatments, another objective was to use essential oils to reduce side effects of interferon and ribavirin and to increase the tolerance to these treatments. Dr. Giraud-Robert reports two case histories for illustration.

Chronic Hepatitis C Treated with Essential Oils Alone

To determine the status of a hepatitis patient the following tests are typically performed.

- Platelet count
- Transaminase levels: SGOT/AST and SGPT/ALT
- Quantitative viral load for hepatitis C, hepatitis B, and eventually HIV if there is co-infection
- Markers of fibrosis and viral activity by biopsy, Fibrotest, or Fibroscan
- Abdominal ultrasound
- Fetoprotein and total serum protein (if there are signs of cirrhosis)
- Complete hepatitis B serology if there is hepatitis B

A seventy-year-old non-insulin-dependent diabetic was described as diagnosed with hepatitis C (genotype 1) in 1995. Her treatment with interferon was stopped after two months because of retinal detachment. Stand-alone essential oil treatment was started in September 2000, because interferon was contraindicated. It was observed that antiviral activity was correlated to the dose of essential oils. As the essential oil dose was increased to three times daily, viral load diminished.

Hepatitis C Treated with Interferon, Ribavirin, and Aromatherapy

A patient aged fifty-three was consulted in December 1999 for her hepatitis C (genotype 1a). Antecedent history included a hysterectomy; the hepatitis C was discovered in 1997. The date of contamination probably dated back to a blood transfusion in 1993. Because of persistently increasing transaminase levels (SGOT at 93 and SFPT at 165) in the beginning of 1999, a standard interferon and ribavirin treatment was proposed to the patient. It began in April 1999, but was stopped by the patient due to very poor tolerance (fatigue and severe depression). During the treatment, transaminase levels normalized. Once interferon was stopped, transaminase levels began to rise rapidly.

Ingesting Revisited: Liver and Prostate

Cultures in South America rely on plant medicine to address imbalances or deficiencies of vital organ systems such as the circulatory system, liver, or the urogenital tract. The anti-infectious qualities of essential oils are fairly well known and have somewhat overshadowed their influence on inner organs and metabolism. Following is a selection of essential oils with distinct activity vis-à-vis liver and prostate!

Greenland Moss

Greenland Moss is a new entry into the circle of commonly used essential oils. Represented in the 1990 edition of *L'aromatherapie exactement,* it has gained larger popularity through Anne-Marie Giraud-Robert's work. She attributes the ability to lower elevated concentrations of transaminase enzymes to this oil. In other words, the essential oil reverses degenerative processes in the liver and restores the integrity of its cell membranes!

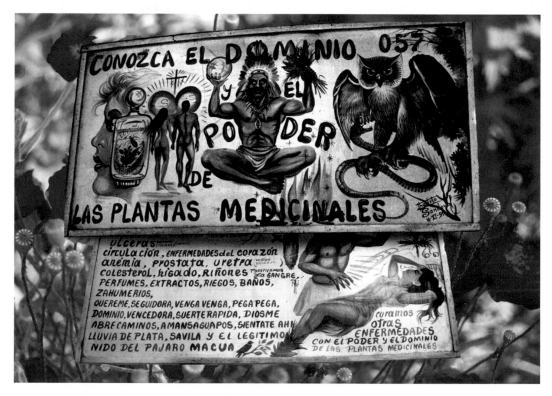

Signage from a medicinal herb stand in the municipal market, Cali, Colombia. The indigenous societies of South America value the healing properties of medicinal plants and are keenly aware of the many ways in which they influence the autonomic nervous system as well as human consciousness.

Carrot Seed

Carrot is credited with liver-regenerating properties across cultures. The essential oil is distilled from the seeds and contains a range of uncommon sesquiterpene components.

Male Issues

There is little experience in aromatherapy with prostate conditions. For those inclined to explore, the following essential oils are listed in *L'aromatherapie exactement* as being related to prostate in one way or another.

Decongestant: *Lentiscus pistachius, Pinus laricio, Cupressus sempervirens, Myrtus communis,* and *Ocimum basilicum*

Inflammation: *Picea mariana, Hypericum perforatum*

At the end of December 1999 the patient began treatment using Greenland Moss, Helichrysum, and Ravintsara essential oils. Already after three weeks of treatment a net reduction in transaminase levels and fatigue was observed. The essential oils effectively normalized transaminase levels, but had little effect on the viral load. Aromatic treatment was followed up regularly over a period of two years. In February 2002, a new treatment with interferon and ribavirin was commenced. At times, the patient used Ravintsara essential oil during her allopathic treatment. This second attempt at allopathic treatment was much better tolerated than the former and ended in February 2003. Tests for hepatitis C virus were negative at the end of treatment as well as six months afterward.

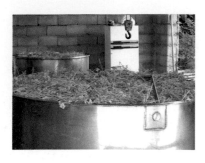

NOTES

Chapter 1. The Foundations of Aromatherapy

1. René-Maurice Gattefossé, *Gattefossé's Aromatherapy* (Saffron Walden, UK: C. W. Daniel Company, 1993).

2. Paul Belaiche, *Traité de phytothérapie et d'aromathérapie* (Paris: Maloine S. A., 1979).

3. J. C. Maruzella, "The Antifungal Properties of Essential Oil Vapors," *Soap, Perfumery and Cosmetics* 33 (1960): 835–37.

4. J. Pellecuer and J. Allegrini, "Place de l'essence de *Satureia montana* L. dans l'arsenal thérapeutique," *Plantes médicinales et phytothérapie* 9, no. 2 (1975): 99–106.

5. V. Jakoviev, O. Issac, K. Thiemer, R. Kunde, "Pharmakologische Untersuchungen von Kamillen Inhaltsstoffen," *Planta Medica* 35, no. 179 (1981): 118–40.

6. A. Lembke and R. Deininger, "Wirkung von Bestandteilen etherischer Öle auf Bakterien, Pilze und Viren," in *Phytotherapie*, ed. H. D. Reuter, R. Deininger, V. Schulz (Stuttgart: Hippokrates, 1988).

7. P. Schnitzler, K. Schön, and J. Reichling, "Antiviral Activity of Australian Tea Tree Oil and Eucalyptus Oil against Herpes Simplex Virus in Cell Culture," *Pharmazie* 56, no. 4 (April 2001): 343–47.

8. H. Wagner and L. Sprinkmeyer, "Über die pharmakologische Wirkung von Melissengeist," *Deutsche Apotheker Zeitung* 113 (1973): 1159–66.

9. A. Sala, M. Recio, R. M. Giner, S. Manez, H. Tournier, G. Schinella, and J. L. Rios, "Anti-inflammatory and Antioxidant Properties of *Helichrysum italicum*," *Journal of Pharmacy and Pharmacology* 54, no. 3 (2002): 365–71.

10. R. Muhlbauer, A. Lozano, S. Palacio, A. Reinli, and R. Felix, "Common Herbs, Essential Oils and Monoterpenes Potently Modulate Bone Metabolism," *Bone* 32, no. 4 (April 2003): 372–80.

11. B. Meier, D. Berger, E. Hoberg, O. Sticher, and W. Schaffner, "Pharmaco-logical Activities of *Vitex agnus-castus* Extracts In Vitro," *Phytomedicine* 7, no. 5 (2000): 373–81.

12. Anne-Marie Giraud-Robert, "The Role of Aromatherapy in the Treatment of Viral Hepatitis," *The International Journal of Aromatherapy* 15 (2005): 183–92.

13. C. E. Elson and S. G. Yu, "The Chemoprevention of Cancer by Mevalonate-derived Constituents of Fruits and Vegetables," *The Journal of Nutrition* 124 (1994): 607–14.

14. Urban Johard, Anders Eklund, Jan Hed, and Joachim Lundahl, "Terpenes Enhance Metabolic Activity and Alter Expression of Adhesion Molecules (Mac-1 and L-selectin) on Human Granulocytes," *Inflammation* 174 (1993): 499–509.

15. Pamela L. Crowell, Charles E. Elson, Howard H. Bailey, Abiodun Elegbede, Jill D. Haag, Michael N. Gould, "Human Metabolism of the Experimental Cancer Therapeutic Agent D-limonene," *Cancer Chemotherapy and Pharmacology* 351 (1994): 31–37.

16. S. P. Hehner et al., "Sesquiterpene Lactones Specifically Inhibit Activation of NF-kappa Beta by Preventing the Degradation of I Kappa B-alpha and I Kappa B-beta," *The Journal of Biological Chemistry* 273 (1998): 1288.

Chapter 2. The Bioactivity of Essential Oils

1. Kurt Schnaubelt, *Biology of Essential Oils* (San Rafael, Calif.: Terra Linda Scent and Image, 2002).

2. E. O. Wilson, *The Diversity of Life* (New York: W. W. Norton & Company, 1999).

Chapter 3. From Biology to Aromatherapy

1. F. Berthou, "Cytochrome P450 Enzyme Regulation by Induction and Inhibition" (lecture series, University of Chile, Santiago de Chile, October 8–12, 2001).

2. Michael Wink, "Evolutionary Advantage and Molecular Modes of Action of Multi-Component Mixtures in Phytomedicine," *Essential Oils, Cancer, Degenerative, and Autoimmune Diseases, Proceedings of the 7th Scientific Aromatherapy Conference,* ed. Kurt Schnaubelt (San Rafael, Calif.: Terra Linda Scent and Image, 2009), 279–318.

Chapter 4. Authentic Essential Oils

1. Cropwatch Newsletter, "Toxicological Imperialism Issue," August 2007, www.cropwatch.org/newsletaug07.pdf.

2. E. Teuscher, M. Melzig, E. Villmann, K. U. Möritz, "Untersuchungen zum Wirkmechanismus ätherischer Öle," *Zeitschrift für Phytotherapie* 113 (1990): 87–92; M. Wink, "Evolutionary Advantage and Molecular Modes of Action of Multi-Component Mixtures in Phytomedicine," *Essential Oils, Cancer, Degenerative, and Autoimmune Diseases, Proceedings of the 7th Scientific Aromatherapy Conference*, ed. Kurt Schnaubelt (San Rafael, Calif.: Terra Linda Scent and Image, 2009), 279–318.

3. Pierre Franchomme and Daniel Pénoël, *L'aromathérapie éxactement* (Limoges, France: Edition Jollois, 1990).

Chapter 5. Aromatherapy Safety

1. D. L. Opdyke, "Monographs on Fragrance Raw Materials," *Food and Cosmetics Toxicology* 11, no. 1 (1973): 95–115.

2. Ron Guba, "Toxicity Myths—The Actual Risks of Essential Oil Use," home.earthlink.net/~skinesscentuals/Toxicity.htm.

3. Kurt Schnaubelt, ed., *Essential Oils and Cancer, Proceedings of the 4th Aromatherapy Conference on the Therapeutic Uses of Essential Oils* (San Rafael, Calif.: Pacific Institute of Aromatherapy, 2000).

4. Kurt Schnaubelt, *Aromatherapy Lifestyle* (San Rafael, Calif.: Terra Linda Scent and Image, 2004).

5. Robert Tisserand, *Essential Oil Safety Data Manual* (Brighton, UK: Aromatherapy Publications, 1988).

6. Kurt Schnaubelt, *Advanced Aromatherapy: The Science of Essential Oil Therapy* (Rochester, Vt.: Healing Arts Press, 1998).

7. Theodore Roszak, *The Cult of Information* (New York: Pantheon, 1986).

8. J. H. Zwaving and R. Bos, "Composition of the Essential Fruit Oil of *Vitex agnus castus,*" *Planta Medica* 62 (1996): 83–84.

9. Kurt Schnaubelt, "Lavender," *Aroma* (San Rafael, Calif.: Terra Linda Scent and Image, 2000): 2–19.

Chapter 6. Aromatherapy Connects with Diverse Traditions

1. Rosemary Caddy, *Essential Oils in Colour* (Guildford, UK: Amberwood Publishing, 1997).
2. H. Reissenweber, "Japanische Phytotherapie (Kampo) und ihr Stellenwert in der modernen Medizin," *Zeitschrift für Phytotherapie* 23 (2002): 242–46.
3. Jeffrey Yuen, *Materia Medica of Essential Oils (Based on a Chinese Medical Perspective)* (Self-published, transcript available from http://www.herbalroom.com/images/stories/jyorder.pdf).

Chapter 7. The Mystery of Fragrance

1. J. S. Jellinek, "Aroma-Chology: A Status Review," *Perfumer & Flavorist* 195 (1994): 25.
2. S. Van Toller and G. H. Dodd, eds., *Perfumery: The Psychology and Biology of Fragrance* (London: Chapman & Hall, 1988); S. Van Toller and G. H. Dodd, eds., *Fragrance: The Psychology and Biology of Perfume* (Essex: Elsevier Science Publishers, 1992).
3. K. Büchner, H. Hellings, M. Huber, E. Peukert, L. Späth, and R. Deininger, "Doppelblindstudie zum Nachweis der therapeutischen Wirkung von Melissengeist bei psychovegetativen Syndromen," *Medizinische Klinik* 69 (1974): 1032–36.
4. John C. Eccles, *The Evolution of the Brain: Creation of the Self* (London: Routledge, 1989).

Chapter 8. How to Apply Essential Oils: Topically

1. Pamela L. Taylor, *Simple Ways of Healing* (Moline, Ill.: MidWest Botanicals, 2007).

Chapter 9. How to Apply Essential Oils: Internally

1. Pierre Franchomme and Daniel Pénoël, *L'aromathérapie éxactement* (Limoges, France: Edition Jollois, 1990).

Chapter 10. Essential Oils for Infections, Allergies, Pain, Insomnia, and Grief

1. David Mitchell, "CDC Interim Guidance Responds to Growing Oseltamivir Resistance in Influenza A (H1N1)," January 22, 2009, www.aafp.org.
2. J. C. Maruzella, "The Antifungal Properties of Essential Oil Vapors," *Soap, Perfumery and Cosmetics* 33 (1960): 835–37.
3. J. Pellecuer and J. Allegrini, "Place de l'essence de *Satureia montana* L. dans l'arsenal thérapeutique," *Plantes Medicinales et Phytothérapie* 9, no. 2 (1975): 99–106.

Chapter 11. Essential Oils and the Skin

1. D. Gümbel, *Ganzheitsmedizinische Hauttherapie mit Heilkräuteressenzen* (Heidelberg, Germany: Haug, 1984).

Chapter 12. Treating Chemotherapy-Induced Vomiting and Nausea

1. Pamela L. Taylor, "Natural Remedies for Chemotherapy-Induced Nausea and Vomiting," *Essential Oils, Cancer, Degenerative, and Autoimmune Diseases, Proceedings of the 7th Scientific Aromatherapy Conference San Francisco,* ed. Kurt Schnaubelt (San Rafael, Calif.: Terra Linda Scent and Image, 2009), 275–94.

Chapter 13. Aromatherapy and Cancer

1. C. E. Myers, J. Trepel, E. Sausville, D. Samid, A. Miller, G. Curt, "Monoterpenes, Sesquiterpenes and Diterpenes as Cancer Therapy," U.S. Patent: 5,602,184 (1997).
2. Charles E. Elson, Dennis M. Peffley, Patricia Hentosh, Huanbiao Mo, "Functional Consequences of Isoprenoid-Mediated Inhibition of Mevalonate Synthesis: Application to Cancer and Cardiovascular Disease," *Essential Oils and Cancer, Proceedings of the 4th Aromatherapy Conference on the Therapeutic Uses of Essential Oils*, ed. Kurt Schnaubelt (San Rafael, Calif.: Pacific Institute of Aromatherapy, 2000), 117–89.

3. Anne-Marie Giraud-Robert, "Essential Oils to Improve Quality of Life During Cancer," 77–118, and "Essential Oils: Effect on Median Survival Rates in Cancer," 119–86, in *Essential Oils, Cancer, Degenerative, and Autoimmune Diseases, Proceedings of the 7th Scientific Aromatherapy Conference,* ed. Kurt Schnaubelt (San Rafael, Calif.: Terra Linda Scent and Image, 2009).
4. P. L. Crowell, "Prevention and Therapy of Cancer by Dietary Monoterpenes," *The Journal of Nutrition* 129 (1999): 775–78.
5. Anne-Marie Giraud-Robert, "Essential Oils to Improve Quality of Life During Cancer," 77–118.

Chapter 14. Selected Aspects of Chinese Medical Aromatherapy: Cancer and Autoimmune Diseases

1. Jeffrey Yuen, *Chinese Medical Aromatherapy* (San Rafael, Calif.: Terra Linda Scent and Image, 2006) (compact disc).

Chapter 15. Essential Oils and Hepatitis B and C

1. Anne-Marie Giraud-Robert, "The Role of Aromatherapy in the Treatment of Viral Hepatitis," *The International Journal of Aromatherapy* 15 (2005): 183–92.

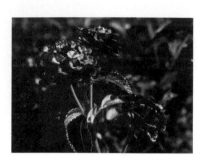

GLOSSARY

Note to the reader: Terms from Chinese medicine have not been entered into the glossary, as representing their meaning most accurately in the English language is not so much a matter of a precise definition as a matter of a translation that reproduces many of the implied meanings of the original Chinese texts.

Also the more specific terms from the work of Dr. Giraud-Robert, while explained in the text, have not been adopted into the glossary, as many of those terms do not appear to be frequently used in the English medical literature, although they are commonly used in French texts in the area of cancer medicine.

1.8 Cineole: A ubiquitous terpenoid essential oil constituent.

acetylcholine: Acetyl ester of choline. A well characterized neurotransmitter, especially on the interface of nerves and muscles.

acid: Water and watery solutions can be alkaline, neutral, or acidic. Acidic refers to the state in which there is an excess of hydrogen ions. This is associated with acidic taste and other features of acids.

Al Andalus: The Arabic name given to the Moorish parts of the Iberian peninsula. Today partly identical with the Spanish region of Andalusia.

alkaline: Water and watery solutions can be alkaline, neutral, or acidic. Alkaline refers to the state in which there is an excess of hydroxyl (OH) ions. Alkalinity makes water soapy to the touch.

alkaloids: Usually refers to biologically active molecules produced by plants. They are historically called alkaloids because they contain nitrogen, which makes the overall molecule (slightly) alkaline.

amino acids: Essential building blocks of many vital biomolecules. Amino acids are characterized by the presence of an amino (NH_2) group (alkaline) and a carboxyl (COOH) group (acidic). As a result amino acids integrate alkaline and acidic functionality (referred to as amphoteric).

amino group: NH_2 functional groups generally impart a more or less alkaline character to a molecule.

amphoteric: Having both alkaline and acidic characteristics. This is one of the defining qualities of amino acids and proteins.

anti-aromatase: Anti-aromatase drugs block the enzyme aromatase which produces estrogen. Used in breast cancer treatments.

antispasmodic: Suppressing muscle spasms.

apoptosis: The most common form of physiological (as opposed to pathological) cell death.

authentic (essential oil): In the context of aromatherapy an authentic essential oil is derived from the plants of one species, ideally from a more or less homogeneous geographical area. No laboratory interventions are applied to the distilled essential oil with the potential exception of filtering or drying (removal of small concentrations of distillation water suspended in the oil).

autonomic nervous system (ANS): Nerve cells not under conscious control, comprising two antagonistic components, the sympathetic and the parasympathetic nervous system. Together they control the heart, the internal organs, smooth muscle, and so on.

biomembrane: An enclosing barrier, generally around or in a cell. It is a selective barrier in that it is permeable to some substances and not so to others.

biotransformation: The chemical modification made to a substance by an organism, typically via the chemical reactions induced by enzymes.

bisabolol: A sesquiterpene alcohol found in the essential oil of German Chamomile (and a number of other plants) with strong anti-inflammative activity.

carbon dioxide (CO_2) extract: So-called supercritical carbon dioxide can be used to obtain plant extracts that are quite similar to the essential oils of the respective plants. However, by changing the parameters of the extraction process, higher molecular components than essential oils can also be extracted. Carbon dioxide will extract polar and nonpolar components from plant materials.

carboxyl: The carboxyl group (-COOH) is the defining structural element of organic acids, for instance, in formic or acetic acid.

carminative: The property of preventing the formation of gas in the intestinal tract.

carotenoids: Lipophilic, photosynthetic pigments in plants. Typically found in the chloroplast, they are products of the terpenoid biosynthetic pathway.

carrier oil: A liquid, cream, or ointment to which essential oils are added.

choleretic: Stimulating bile production by the liver.

chromatography (chromatogram): Testing technique (and result) that separates the molecules of a mixture, by methods involving the flow of a fluid carrier over a nonmobile absorbing phase.

conformation: The shape or three-dimensional structure of a protein.

covalent (bond): The chemical bond between two atoms that is mediated by a pair of electrons.

cyclooxygenase (COX): Enzymes present in most tissues producing various prostaglandins (and thromboxanes from arachidonic acid). These enzymes are inhibited by aspirin-like drugs!

CYP (cytochrome P 450): CYP is a short notation for cytochrome P 450, a large group of oxidative enzymes with a variety of functions. Besides detoxifying xenobiotics they also remove endogenous substances such as hormones.

cytokine: Small proteins released from cells, which affect the behavior of other cells. The term tends to be used as a shorthand for interleukins, lymphokines, and signaling molecules like TNF or interferons.

cytotoxic: Toxic to the cell.

decongestant: A decongestant is a drug that relieves congestion. While most decongestant drugs work by enhancing noradrenaline or adrenaline or by stimulating adrenergic receptors, it is unclear whether decongestant essential oils work by the same mechanism.

diketones: Literally a molecule with two ketone groups. These molecules have a tendency to be present in a form where one ketone group remains and the other rearranges into a hydroxyl group.

diterpene: Common component of essential oils; a volatile unsaturated hydrocarbon with 20 carbon atoms. *See* **terpenes.**

DNA: Deoxyribonucleic acid. The genetic material of all cells and many viruses.

dopamine: A neurotransmitter and hormone.

endorphins: A family of peptide hormones that bind to receptors that mediate the actions of opiates.

enzyme: A protein that catalyzes chemical reactions.

ester: The reaction (condensation) product arising from an alcohol and an acid under loss of one molecule of water.

farnesene: Sesquiterpene hydrocarbon, frequently present in floral essential oils such as German Chamomile, Ylang Ylang, or Rose.

fibrosis: Deposition of a collagen rich matrix (fibrous tissue) usually as a consequence of extensive tissue damage as in sites of chronic inflammation.

Fine Lavender: The term used by growers and the trade in Provence to describe population Lavender.

flavonoids: A class of plant secondary metabolites or yellow pigments. The basic structure is that of 2-phenyl-1, 4-benzopyrone.

functional protein: An umbrella term summarizing all types of proteins that perform functions in the cell, such as enzymes, neurotransmitters, or receptors.

GABA: Gamma amino butyric acid. Fast neurotransmitter in the mammalian central nervous system.

galactose: A sugar similar to glucose. A component of gangliosides, lipids found in high concentration in nerve cells.

gamma GT: Gamma-glutamyltransferase (GGT) is an enzyme that plays a key role in the gamma-glutamyl cycle, a pathway for the synthesis and degradation of glutathione and drug and xenobiotic detoxification.

GC-MS: Gas chromatography linked with mass spectrometry. In the chromatography step a mixture is separated into its components. The isolated components enter the mass spectrometer where they are identified as a consequence of their molecular mass (weight) and their fragmentation patterns.

gene expression: The full use of the information in a gene via transcription and translation leading to the production of a protein and hence the appearance of the quality of the gene is coding for (phenotype). For the phenomena of secondary metabolites it is relevant that not all genes are always expressed; they may be present but remain unutilized.

genotype: The genetic constitution of an organism or cell, as distinct from its expressed features (phenotype).

genuine and authentic: The term introduced by Henri Viaud to describe essential oils not subjected to the various engineering processes of the flavor and fragrance industry. In this book also simply referred to as "authentic."

geraniol: A common monoterpene alcohol, especially prevalent in essential oil of Palmarosa or *Monarda fistulosa*.

H1N1: Influenza A (H1N1) virus is a subtype of influenza A virus and was the most common cause of human influenza (flu) in 2009. Some strains of H1N1 are endemic in humans. Other strains of H1N1 are endemic in pigs (swine influenza) and in birds (avian influenza).

hepatitis: Inflammation of the liver. Commonly caused by infection with hepatitis virus type A or B.

herbivore: An organism that eats plants.

Glossary

213

histamine: Strong agent triggering inflammatory responses through receptors in smooth muscle and secretory systems.

HMG CoA reductase: This integral membrane protein (enzyme) catalyzes a reaction of hydroxymethylglutaryl CoA to produce mevalonate. Mevalonate leads to isoprene and isoprene to monoterpenes, representing the first steps in the synthesis of cholesterol. Because this enzyme limits the rate of cholesterol synthesis it has been identified as a target for cholesterol-lowering drugs such as statins.

hydrophilic: Water soluble. *See* BioPrimer.

hydrophobic: Water repelling. Not soluble in water.

hypothyroidism: Hypothyroidism is a condition in which the thyroid gland does not make enough thyroid hormone. Symptoms include being more sensitive to cold, constipation, depression, fatigue, or feeling slowed down.

interferon: A family of glycoproteins produced in mammals that prevent virus multiplication in cells.

ketone: Basic structural element in which oxygen is bound to carbon by a double bond.

ligand: Any molecule that binds to another. In common usage, a hormone or neurotransmitter that binds to a receptor.

limonene: Common monoterpene hydrocarbon present in many essential oils.

linalool: Common monoterpene alcohol present in many essential oils.

linalyl acetate: Common ester formed from the alcohol linalool and acetic acid.

lipids: Biological molecules soluble in nonpolar solvents. They are a heterogeneous group, defined only on the basis of solubility.

lipophilic: Oily or oil soluble, water insoluble.

mitochondria: Organelle of eukaryotic cells with highly variable structure. Their inner fluid phase contains many enzymes and their major function is to regenerate ATP (adenosine triphosphate) by oxidative phosphorylation.

monoterpenes: Common component of essential oils; a volatile unsaturated hydrocarbon with 10 carbon atoms. *See* **terpenes.**

mucositis: Inflammation of the mucous membranes.

nature identical: The term is mostly used in the field of flavor and fragrance and is applied to food additives that are synthesized in the laboratory and are considered identical to those that occur in nature, because superficially they have the same structural formula as their natural counterparts.

nervine: A nerve tonic, acting on the nerves, generally in the sense of a sedative that calms ruffled nerves.

neuraminidase: A transmembrane protein of the envelope of the influenza virus.

neurotransmitter: Substance found in chemical synapses (the connection between two excitable cells), crucial for transduction of electric signals. Examples: acetylcholine, GABA, noradrenaline, serotonin, dopamine.

neutral: Water and watery solutions can be alkaline, neutral, or acidic. Neutral refers to the state in which there are an equal number of hydrogen and hydroxyl ions.

neutropenia: Condition in which the number of neutrophils (the most common blood leucocyte responsible for primary response to acute inflammation) circulating in the blood is below normal.

nonpolar: When electrons are equally shared in the chemical bonds of a molecule, making it insoluble in water but soluble in oil.

noradrenaline: Also called norepinephrine. Neurotransmitter of most of the sympathetic nervous system.

nucleus: The major organelle of eukaryotic cells in which the chromosomes are separated from the cytoplasm.

organelle: A structurally discrete area of the cell, housing specific physiological processes.

organicism: One of the fundamental doctrines of contemporary biology, which holds that within the organizational hierarchy of living organisms (emergent) properties arise at each level of organization.

paracymene: A common monoterpene found in essential oils.

perillyl alcohol: Terpene alcohol derived from Limonene. Occurs in higher concentration in the essential oil of Yuzu. Also a metabolite of Phase I oxidation of Limonene in the liver.

phenylpropanoids: Found throughout the plant kingdom, phenylpropanoids serve as essential components of a number of structural polymers. Among other things phenylpropanoid derivatives, such as floral pigments and scent compounds, provide protection from ultraviolet light, defend against herbivores and pathogens, and mediate plant-pollinator interactions. Phenylpropanes are distinguished by their biosynthetic origin, ultimately arising from amino acid synthesis in the chloroplast.

phospholipid: The major structural lipid of most cellular membranes (except the chloroplast, which has galactolipids).

photosynthesis: Process by which green plants and green algae absorb light energy and use it to synthesize organic compounds. In green plants this process occurs in chloroplasts, which contain the photosynthetic pigments.

physicalism: The thesis that the nature of the universe and everything in it conforms to the condition of being physical. Physicalists don't deny that the world might contain phenomena that at first glance don't seem physical—phenomena of a biological, psychological, moral, or social nature. But they insist nevertheless that ultimately such items are either physical or caused by the physical.

platelet: Disk-like cells found in blood, important for coagulation and hemostasis.

pleiotropic: Having multiple effects. Used in this book mainly to describe the multiple effects of secondary metabolites. An example other than secondary metabolites in the cell would be cyclo-AMP, which has a variety of effects on intracellular signaling.

polar: When the electrons in a chemical bond are not shared equally. This results in increased solubility in water.

population Lavender: Lavender grown from seed as opposed to being grown from clipped (cloned) branches.

primary metabolites (or primary plant substances): All those components that comprise the bulk of the biomass and basically perform a plant's daily activities. They are proteins, carbohydrates, fats and oils, and genetic materials such as DNA.

protein: A polymer of amino acids in a specific sequence.

receptor: A membrane-bound or membrane-enclosed molecule that responds to mobile molecules, typically called ligands, with great specificity.

reductionism: Reductionism is currently the most broadly accepted paradigm of scientific methodology. Complex phenomena are explained by parsing them down to ever smaller components and then analyzing the simplest, most basic physical mechanisms present in the phenomenon.

RNA: Ribonucleic acid. Plays an informational, structural, and enzymatic role in the cell.

ROS: Reactive oxygen species. Oxygen-containing reactive species, responsible for killing pathogenic bacteria but also for incidental damage to surrounding tissue.

salicylic acid: Salicylic acid historically was obtained from the bark of the willow tree (e.g. *Salix alba*). It functions as a plant hormone. It served as the primary structure that was modified to result in acetyl salicylic acid, one of the most common analgesic drugs. In the plant, salicylic acid ultimately arises from the same biosynthetic path as do the phenylpropanoids.

scleroderma: Scleroderma is a widespread connective tissue disease that involves changes in the skin, blood vessels, muscles, and internal organs.

secondary metabolites: Substances that are spun off the biosynthetic pathways that manufacture primary metabolites, and then, coincidentally, help the survival of the plant, for instance by repelling herbivores. Over time these substances became not only the defense mechanism but also the communication system of the plant. Essential oils are one large group of secondary plant metabolites.

semisynthetic: Semisynthetic in the context of essential oils typically refers to components that came originally from plants but have been isolated and then altered by chemical reactions.

sensitization: Heightened responsiveness of the immune system after a primary challenge. In other words, a status that leads to an unexpectedly strong response to renewed exposure to an allergen, even if the contact is only with minute concentrations.

serotonin: A neurotransmitter and hormone found in vertebrates, invertebrates, and plants.

sesquiterpenes: Common component of essential oils; a volatile unsaturated hydrocarbon with a structure made up from 15 carbon atoms. *See* **terpenes**.

sesquiterpene lactone: A large group of physiologically active sesquiterpene derivatives. Lactone refers to a structural element where an ester is formed within a single molecule, resulting in a ring structure.

spasmolytic: Providing relief from cramping, spasms, and convulsions.

terpenes: A large group of volatile unsaturated hydrocarbons, found in the essential oils of plants. These organic compounds are major biosynthetic building blocks within nearly every living creature. They are distinguished by their biosynthetic origin from the terpenoid cholesterol synthetic pathway. Terpenes may be classified by the number of terpene units in the molecule, indicated by a prefix in the name, giving rise to monoterpenes, diterpenes, sesquiterpenes, and so on.

thrombopenia: A blood disease characterized by an abnormally small number of platelets in the blood.

thujone: Monoterpene ketone occurring in Thuja and Sage essential oils, among others.

thuyanol: Terpene alcohol with specific effects against chlamydia and which promotes liver regeneration.

transaminase: Enzymes that convert amino acids to keto acids.

vegetative symptoms: Symptoms caused by imbalances of the autonomic (or vegetative) nervous system; for instance, loss of appetite or insomnia.

verbenone: A monoterpene ketone, best known for its occurrence in Rosemary essential oils.

vitalism: The thesis that living organisms are fundamentally different from nonliving entities because they contain some nonphysical element or are governed by different principles than are inanimate things.

volatile: Molecules that are volatile easily evaporate under ambient conditions.

xenobiotic: Any substance foreign to an organism.

RECOMMENDED READING

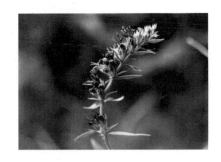

The works that pertain to the more technical subject matter of this book are listed in the notes section and are not repeated here. The writings listed here are mostly those from outside the realm of aromatherapy, which nonetheless had a strong impact as I was forming the ideas for *The Healing Intelligence of Essential Oils.* The books listed here are intended to serve as a guide for the reader who wishes to explore the universe that unfolds at the interface between human culture and plant secondary metabolites.

Bartholomew, Terese Tse. *Hidden Meaning in Chinese Art.* San Francisco: The Asian Art Museum, 2006. This was published on the occasion of the exhibition of the same title. It is a comprehensive representation of how plants and animals acquired their symbolic meaning in Chinese culture.

Berry, Wendell. *Life Is a Miracle.* Washington D.C.: Counterpoint, 2000. A most beautiful essay in response to E. O. Wilsons's *Consilience.* It addresses the issues of plant, animal, and human life not through abstract data but through the eyes of the heart.

Bingen, Hildegard. *Physica.* Augsburg: Pattloch, 1997. The first time Hildegard's writings have been published in their original, unabridged version.

Bloßfeldt, Karl. *Das Photographische Werk.* Munich: Schirmer und Mosel, 1981. Another glorious result of human fascination with the plant world: plant photography in fascinating detail from the beginning of the twentieth century.

Haas, Monika. *Quick Reference Guide to 114 Essential Oils.* San Rafael, Calif.: Terra Linda Scent and Image, 2004. Short and precise essential oil facts.

Haeckel, Ernst. *Art Forms in Nature.* Munich: Prestel, 1998. An epic work, which captures, in the words of its author, nature's "sense of the beautiful." Brilliant art revealing the diversity and complexity of many minuscule organisms!

Keay, John. *The Spice Route: A History.* Berkeley: California University Press, 2006. A riveting literary journey through space and time to the earliest origins of the spice trade. An unwitting account of the power of plant secondary metabolites.

Mayr, Ernst. *This Is Biology.* Boston: Belknap Press/Harvard University Press, 1997. An introduction to the science of biology from one of its most renowned protagonists. An indispensable resource for anyone who feels that the current mechanistic and chemistry-centered paradigm has monopolized the discourse on health and healing far beyond its capacity to provide meaningful answers.

Raven, Peter H., Ray F. Evert, and Susan E. Eichhorn. *Biology of Plants.* New York: W. H. Freeman, 1999. The current textbook of botany; despite its academic scope it offers great appeal to the lay reader.

Roszak, Theodore. *The Cult of Information.* New York: Pantheon Books, 1986. If one wonders whether ever more aspects of our lives need to be run by digital devices, this treatise argues that this slide into an information economy has been carefully planned and executed since the end of World War II.

Schnaubelt, Kurt. *Biology of Essential Oils.* San Rafael, Calif.: Terra Linda Scent and Image, 2002. This part of the PIA (Pacific Institute of Aromatherapy) Masters Series offers a glimpse at the research exploring the interactions between plant secondary metabolites and human physiological systems.

Schnaubelt, Kurt, ed. *Essential Oils and Cancer, Proceedings of the 4th Aromatherapy Conference on the Therapeutic Uses of Essential Oils.* San Rafael, Calif.: Terra Linda Scent and Image, 2000. A direct entry into the antitumor effects of essential oil components, especially terpenoids.

Schnaubelt, Kurt, ed. *Essential Oils, Cancer, Degenerative, and Autoimmune Diseases, Proceedings of the 7th Scientific Aromatherapy Conference San Francisco.* San Rafael, Calif.: Terra Linda Scent and Image, 2009. Includes many outstanding contributions to the most recent PIA conference, including original papers by Prof. Franzblau (essential oil activity vis-à-vis tuberculosis) and Dr. Anne-Marie Giraud-Robert (on essential oils in cancer therapy).

Schnaubelt, Kurt. *Medical Aromatherapy.* Berkeley: North Atlantic Books, 1999. Provides a perspective toward the healing qualities of essential oils that recognizes that plant activity is independent of commercial and corporate directives.

Taylor, Pamela L. *Simple Ways of Healing.* Moline, Ill.: Midwest Botanicals, 2007. A comprehensive guide that turns the theory into practical applications.

Tompkins, Peter, and Christopher Bird. *The Secret Life of Plants.* New York: Harper & Row, 1973. What was considered somewhat puzzling and outlandish thirty years ago reveals a deep understanding of plant life when viewed through the lens of organicism.

Virilio, Paul. *The Art of the Motor.* Minneapolis: University of Minnesota Press, 1996. Virilio describes the gradual takeover of the human body by the forces of technology and commerce. Giving in to the temptations of ever more plastic (or other) surgery and mechanization and digitization of vital functions explains why we, as a society, lose interest in nature.

Wilson, E. O. *The Diversity of Life.* New York: W.W. Norton & Company, 1999. The *New York Times* called it the "best selling celebration of the miracle of evolution."

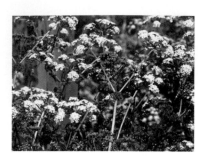

RESOURCES

With essential oils as with many other precious natural materials, the truly exquisite specimens are always sought after and in relatively short supply while their allure is co-opted and attached to the not-so-exquisite products so that these can sell better by absorbing some of the glory of the original. As a consequence, it is with essential oils as with, for instance, fine wine: there is plenty to go around but only a small fraction is truly the very best.

Dealing in authentic essential oils can be a frustrating experience, as time and again the price of a truly authentic oil is compared to that of its industrial brethren. The business of trading in authentic oils is essentially characterized by always being in competition, not with other vendors of authentic oils, but rather with those dealing in industrial products. Even for individuals with experience in purchasing essential oils, the price differentials between authentic and industrial are hard to rationalize. We are so accustomed to comparing prices, and the lower price will generally be the better deal because so often they are for identical products. The difficulty with authentic essential oils is that identical names give the impression that we are comparing prices of identical products, but we are not. There is a world of difference between those Lavender oils that come out of seemingly inexhaustible barrels and are available at rather modest prices and those that are distilled from hand-gathered plants from the high plateaus of Provence.

This is the reason that my list of recommendations for essential oil resources is rather short. The operators of the businesses dealing in authentic essential oils have chosen to forgo the economic growth potential vested in industrial essential oils in favor of the quality of life that results from being surrounded by authentic oils.

And while it is hard to guarantee that 100 percent of all the oils of a specific company are authentic, it is my experience that the businesses mentioned on the following pages go to extreme lengths to offer their clients what in the context of this book is called authentic essential oils.

Resources for Authentic Essential Oils

Essential Therapeutics: Ron Guba
39 Mclverton Drive
Hallam, VICTORIA 3803
Australia
phone: 03 8795 7720
fax: 03 8795 7375
www.essentialtherapeutics.com

Ron has been the pioneer of the French style of aromatherapy in Australia.

Laboratory of Flowers: Michael Scholes
21010 Southbank Street #630
Sterling, VA 20165
phone: (703) 433-2499
fax: (310) 388-5841
www.labofflowers.com

Michael has been a most outstanding ambassador for aromatherapy for decades.

Nature's Gift: Marge Clark
316 Old Hickory Blvd. East
Madison, TN 37115
fax: (615) 860-9171
www.naturesgift.com

Offers a wide range of essential oils and myriad other products.

Original Swiss Aromatics: Kurt Schnaubelt and Monika Haas
P.O. Box 6842
San Rafael, CA 94903
phone: (415) 479-9120
fax: (415) 479-0614
www.originalswissaromatics.com

Has a range of approximately 130 essential oils with a focus on specialties from small French distillers and hard-to-find medicinal rarities. In addition, OSA offers a collection of all the essential oils mentioned in the journey sections of this book.

White Lotus Aromatics: Christopher and Suzanne McMahon
602 S. Alder Street
Port Angeles, WA 98362-6614
fax: (360) 457-9235
e-mail: somanath@aol.com
www.whitelotusaromatics.com

Offers a wide range of authentic essential oils from all over the world with absolutes and extracts of some of the most precious natural fragrances, especially those from India.

Aromatherapy Education and Learning

There is a wide range of offerings available for aromatherapy education and seminars, differing significantly in style and substance. The following individuals and schools are mentioned because their style and content have emerged from French-style aromatherapy origins, emphasizing knowledge of the essential oils.

Suzanne Catty

www.suzannecatty.com

Suzanne is an aromatherapy teacher who brings her experience as a practicing therapist to the field. She has contributed to the field immensely, and her style and approach can be sampled in her book *Hydrosols: The Next Aromatherapy.*

London School of Aromatherapy (LSA), Tokyo: Ayako Berg
6-18-11-4F, Akasaka
Minato-ku
Tokyo 107-0052
Japan
phone/fax: 813-6426-5068
e-mail: contact@lsajapan.com
www.lsajapan.com

Under the direction of Ayako Berg, the London School of Aromatherapy in Tokyo, Japan, offers some of the most advanced and in-depth courses in the style of aromatherapy presented in this book.

Quantum Aromatherapy: Daniel Pénoël

www.osmobiose.com

www.ecolepenoel.com

e-mail: ecolepenoel@orange.fr

Dr. Pénoël's Quantum Aromatherapy integrates French-style aromatherapy, medical aromatherapy, and Quantum physics. Osmobiose and l'Ecole Pénoël in France (see websites above) offer workshops in Europe and throughout the world. Books and other products are also available through the websites.

Pacific Institute of Aromatherapy (PIA): Kurt Schnaubelt and Monika Haas

P.O. Box 6723

San Rafael, CA 94903

phone: (415) 479-9121

fax: (415) 479 0614

www.pacificinstituteofaromatherapy.com

www.plantlanguage.org

PIA offers distance learning, seminars, and conferences as well as publications and tours to essential oil producers.

There are currently three different distance learning programs offered. **The Aromatherapy Correspondence Course** is a classic introduction to French-style aromatherapy, exploring the therapeutic effects of essential oils based on an understanding of the pharmacology of their chemical components. This course was established in 1985 and is one of the most studied in the United States.

Following completion of the basic correspondence course, students may take the more in-depth **PIA Masters Series,** which is based on the study of three texts: *The Chemistry of Essential Oils, The Biology of Essential Oils,* and *Aromatherapy Lifestyle.*

The Plant Language Course is different from all other aromatherapy courses in that it focuses not so much on setting up a practice as on building a personal body of experience with the essential oils. With this course, the student receives all of the oils from the Essential Oil Journeys provided in this book, making it easy to experience the unique effects of each of these authentic oils.

Also available from PIA are volumes of the proceedings of the scientific aromatherapy conferences that the institute has organized since 1995. These proceedings are a vast repository of information, covering the most diverse aspects of aromatherapy—from strictly academic research to reports from practitioners to the more esoteric aspects.

INDEX

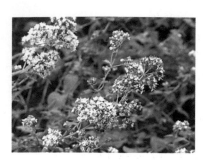

Page numbers in *italics* refer to images.

Books of Related Interest

Advanced Aromatherapy
The Science of Essential Oil Therapy
by Kurt Schnaubelt, Ph.D.

Medical Herbalism
The Science and Practice of Herbal Medicine
by David Hoffmann, FNIMH, AHG

The Encyclopedia of Healing Points
The Home Guide to Acupoint Treatment
by Roger Dalet, M.D.

Aromatherapy for Healing the Spirit
Restoring Emotional and Mental Balance with Essential Oils
by Gabriel Mojay

The Art of Aromatherapy
The Healing and Beautifying Properties of the Essential Oils of Flowers and Herbs
by Robert B. Tisserand

Hydrosols
The Next Aromatherapy
by Suzanne Catty

Bach Flower Therapy
Theory and Practice
by Mechthild Scheffer

The Encyclopedia of Bach Flower Therapy
by Mechthild Scheffer

INNER TRADITIONS • BEAR & COMPANY
P.O. Box 388
Rochester, VT 05767
1-800-246-8648
www.InnerTraditions.com

Or contact your local bookseller